Building Your Health Care Career:

A Guide for Students

Building Your Health Care Career

A Guide for Students

JANICE WADDELL, RN, PhD

GAIL J. DONNER, RN, PhD

MARY M. WHEELER, RN, MEd, PCC

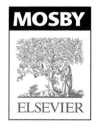

MOSBY

ELSEVIER

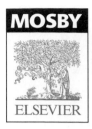

Library and Archives Canada Cataloguing in Publication
Waddell, Janice, 1955–
    Building your health care career: a guide for students / Janice Waddell,
Gail J. Donner, Mary M. Wheeler.
ISBN 978-1-897422-17-5
    1. Allied health personnel – Vocational guidance. I. Donner,
Gail J. (Gail Judith), 1942– II. Wheeler, Mary M. III. Title.
R697.A4W33 2008   610.73'7069   C2008-904619-6

VP, Publishing: Ann Millar
Managing Developmental Editor: Martina van de Velde
Managing Production Editor: Rohini Herbert
Copy Editor: Michael Peebles
Cover Design: Gary Holgate
Interior Design: Monica Kompter
Typesetting and Assembly: Jansom
Printing and Binding: Transcontinental

Elsevier Canada
905 King Street West, 4th Floor
Toronto, ON, Canada M6K 3G9
Phone: 1-866-896-3331
Fax: 1-866-359-9534

Printed in Canada

1 2 3 4 5   13 12 11 10 09

Contents

1 Career Planning and Development as a Student Activity, 1

How to Use *Building Your Health Care Career*, 2
Career Planning and Development, 3
Why Career Planning and Development Is Important for Health Profession Students, 4
The Donner-Wheeler Career Planning and Development Model, 5

2 Planning Your Career, 7

Creating Your Career Vision, 7
What Is a Career Vision?, 7
Why Should You Have a Career Vision?, 8
How to Create Your Own Career Vision, 10
Activity 1: Creating Your Career Vision, 13
What Have You Accomplished?, 16

Scanning Your Environment, 16
What Is Scanning?, 16
Why Is Scanning Important?, 17
How and When Do You Scan?, 17
Activity 2: Scanning Your Environment, 20
What Have You Accomplished?, 25
What Is Your Next Step?, 25

Completing Your Self-Assessment, 25
What Is Self-Assessment?, 25
Why Is Assessing Yourself Important?, 26
Beginning the Self-Assessment Process, 26
Activity 3: Completing Your Self-Assessment, 34
Your Reality Check, 42
Activity 4: Reality Check, 44
What Have You Accomplished?, 46
What Is Your Next Step?, 46

Developing Your Strategic Career Plan, 46

What Is a Career Plan?, 46

Why Should You Develop a Career Plan?, 46

How Should You Plan?, 47

Activity 5: Developing Your Strategic Career Plan, 51

Thinking of Graduate Studies?, 52

What Have You Accomplished?, 53

What Is Your Next Step?, 53

Marketing Yourself, 53

Health Profession Students as Self-Marketers, 53

Why Marketing Yourself Is Important, 54

How Can You Market Yourself?, 54

Activity 6: Marketing Yourself, 64

What Have You Accomplished?, 66

What Next?, 66

(3) Choosing Your First Job as a Health Care Professional, 67

Your Career Vision, 67

Your Environmental Scan, 67

Your Self-Assessment, 68

Your Strategic Career Plan, 69

Marketing, 69

(4) Do You Need More Help?, 70

Appendix A Student Résumés, 71

Generic Student Résumé, 71

Résumé of a Graduating Student Seeking First Health Care Position in a Mental Health Care Setting, 73

Appendix B Graduating Student Cover Letter, 76

Career Planning and Development Resources: A Selected Reading List, 77

About the Authors

Janice Waddell, RN, PhD, is an Associate Professor at The Daphne Cockwell School of Nursing, Ryerson University, Toronto, Ontario. She is currently the Associate Dean for the Faculty of Community Services at Ryerson. Janice's clinical expertise is in the area of child and family violence. Her research foci include career planning and development for nurses (with a particular emphasis on student nurses and nursing faculty), the health experience of aggressive children, and children who have witnessed family violence. She teaches in both the undergraduate and graduate nursing programs at Ryerson University, focusing on advanced nursing education and professional issues and trends. Janice has facilitated numerous student-focused career planning and development workshops across Canada. She has been an Associate of **donnerwheeler** since 1994.

Gail J. Donner, RN, PhD, is a partner in **donnerwheeler**, a consulting company focusing on career planning and development for health care professionals and health care organizations. Gail is a Professor and Dean Emeritus of the Lawrence S. Bloomberg Faculty of Nursing, University of Toronto, and active in nursing, in health care, and in her community.

Mary M. Wheeler, RN, MEd, PCC, is the other half of the **donnerwheeler** partnership. Mary is a certified coach with over 15 years of consulting expertise in career, organization, and human resource development and has published extensively with Gail in the area of career development, coaching, and mentoring.

Career Planning and Development as a Student Activity

Welcome to *Building Your Health Care Career: A Guide for Students*. This guide is intended to provide you with the skills you need to build your career as a health care professional. The rapidly changing world of health care offers tremendous opportunities as well as significant challenges to students. Students now learn in a variety of professional practice settings and thus get a first-hand look at health care professionals who work alone, with others in their profession, or in interprofessional teams in various roles. Changes in the health care system have created an environment in which individuals must become career resilient and self-directed and take control of their careers and futures. Developing the skills necessary for career resilience is a process that students in the health professions should engage in as soon as they begin their education.

Career resilience is about flexibility and adaptability. As a career-resilient student, you seek and take advantage of meaningful and career-enhancing experiences both in the classroom and in your field placement settings.* You develop a growing sense of who you are as a professional and are able to develop incrementally as you move through your educational program. Career-resilient students are dedicated to the idea of continuous learning and stand ready to re-invent themselves to keep pace with change. Moreover, career resilience embodies many characteristics of a health care professional, including autonomy, self-direction, and continual learning. Just as health care professionals share many characteristics, they also share common professional competencies. In this book, the term "competency" refers to "a behaviour or set of behaviours that describes excellent performance in a particular professional context" (Verma, Paterson, & Medves, 2006, p. 109). Health care professional competencies include knowledge, clinical skills (assessment, intervention, evaluation), interpersonal skills, teamwork, problem solving, clinical judgement, and technical skills (Verma et al., 2006).

As a student, you may be exposed to a wide range of professional settings, and you will learn about many current theoretical and technological advances as well as cur-

---

*Many health care profession program curricula include learning experiences outside of academic institutions, in clinics, hospitals, community centres, and other settings that are practice based. These experiences are frequently referred to as field placements, practice settings, practicums, internships, or residencies, depending on the discipline or curriculum. For ease of reading, the term "field placement" will be used to represent all of the experiences that involve student learning and the application of learning in the context of a professional practice setting.

rent health care system issues. In the midst of all your discoveries, it is often easy to lose sight of the career goals and aspirations that brought you to your chosen profession. You may need and want help in planning and developing your career so that you can orchestrate, rather than merely accumulate, your learning experiences.

How can I plan my career? What are the opportunities today, and what will they be in the future? How can I best use my educational experiences to advance my career goals? How can I be employable 1 year or several years from now? Who can help me? These are the questions health profession students are asking. You are coming to your chosen profession with dreams, goals, and ideas about your future. You need a process to guide you in achieving your maximum potential as a student so that you can actualize your dreams or alter them in response to your growing experience and professional identification. Career planning and development is a dynamic process that adapts to the changes you will encounter as you build your professional knowledge and experience.

The purposes of *Building Your Health Care Career* are (1) to enhance your awareness of career planning and development and its importance today and in the future, and (2) to introduce you to a career planning and development model and a variety of career planning and development activities you can use throughout your career. We hope you find this guide to be informative and useful.

HOW TO USE
BUILDING YOUR HEALTH CARE CAREER

Building Your Health Care Career introduces you to the Donner-Wheeler Career Planning and Development Model, referred to from now on as "the Model" (Figure 1–1). This Model is a tool you can use throughout your education to develop as a professional and build your career in a meaningful way. Each phase of the Model (scanning, assessing, visioning, planning, and marketing) is described along with specific activities and exercises to help you develop the skill to use the Model at all points in your educational program and later through the other stages of your career. You can use the Model to select courses, determine foci for course assignments, engage in extracurricular activities, and (most importantly) experience a sense of control over your academic career. Try to encourage your student colleagues to work together as you engage in the career planning and development process. As peers, you can offer each other support, feedback, and affirmation as you build your careers.

If you are a nursing student and want to learn more about using the Model to guide your academic career in nursing, you can read *Building Your Nursing Career: A Guide for Students*, Third Edition (Waddell, Donner, & Wheeler, 2009).

Your first step should be to read about each phase of the Model—what it is, why it is important, and how to use it. Then turn to the activities at the end of the sec-

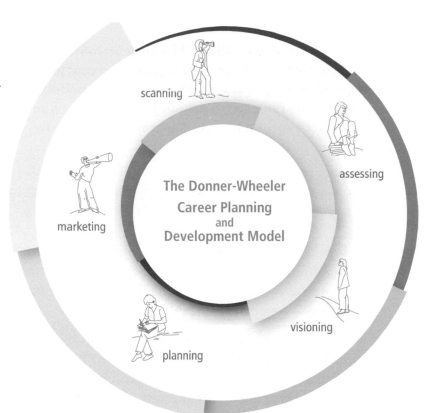

FIGURE 1–1
The Donner-Wheeler Career Planning and Development Model.

tion on each phase and complete the questions. Each activity will help you tailor the career building process to your own situation. As you become comfortable with the process, you will be able to move back and forth with ease among the five phases as you gather new experiences, skills, and knowledge.

Building Your Health Care Career is primarily for students in entry-level health profession programs. As you begin the career planning and development process, you may wish to consider developing an electronic portfolio ("e-portfolio") to record your career planning and development activities. A portfolio can also help you reflect on your career achievements and successes as you work with the Model over the course of your academic program. An e-portfolio is technology based and can contain a significant amount of diverse information, including pictures, artwork, text, sound, video, and creative graphics. If you are not familiar with e-portfolios, you can use the Internet to explore this concept and various ways to develop your professional Web portfolio (e-portfolio) by using a search engine such as Google and typing the search term "e-portfolio" or "web portfolio."

CAREER PLANNING AND DEVELOPMENT

A career is described as one's chosen profession, path, or course of life work. Students often think that their career as a health care professional starts at the completion of their educational program and that active involvement in career planning becomes important only as they near graduation. In fact, you have chosen a path; your career has already started! You made an important life decision and began your professional career the day you registered for your program courses. The career planning and development model presented in this book provides you with a process by which you can develop your unique career goals and influence your educational activities to help you succeed in achieving your goals—regardless of where you are in your program.

WHY CAREER PLANNING AND DEVELOPMENT IS IMPORTANT FOR HEALTH PROFESSION STUDENTS

Health profession students are at various stages of entering a profession that offers incredibly diverse opportunities for professional practice. Students describe feeling both excited and anxious when faced with the range of possibilities open to them. As John, a fourth-year pharmacy student, observed:

> I am currently completing a very important phase of my life by graduating. At the same time, I will be entering one of the most exciting phases by officially starting a career as a pharmacist. What I am realizing is that I am the only one responsible for my career. Opportunities will not simply fall into my hands; rather, I need to take charge and control my professional future through career planning. I know there are lots of jobs out there; I want to make sure I accept a job that is right for me and fits with my career plans.

Although at a different level in her health profession program, Leah, a second-year student, described similar feelings:

> I've just finished the second year of my 4-year program, and I feel like I now have only 2 years left to make sure I get all of the experience I can to be marketable when I graduate. I'm not sure what my goals are or how I can "work the system" to make sure I get what I need.

The career planning process can serve as a guide to help students achieve a sense of control and focus related to their educational activities and to prepare for future employment. The career planning and development process helps students answer the following questions:

✦ Where have I been (prior to my health profession education and over the course of my program)?
✦ Where am I now? What am I learning, and what are my interests?
✦ Where would I like to go? What are my hopes for the next step in my education and for my future career?
✦ How will I get there? How can I plan my courses and make the best of other experiences such as field placements or volunteer work so that I can move toward my goals?

JOHN Over the course of his education, John (the fourth-year student) accumulated a solid foundation of experiences and professional courses. As a result, his responses to these questions will reflect a wide range of discipline-related knowledge and experience.

LEAH Leah (the second-year student) may not have the same breadth of experience and range of course work as John, but she can build on her beginning foundation in her profession, her life experiences, and her hopes and dreams for her professional education. Reflecting on these questions can help Leah acknowledge all that she has brought to her profession and how her education can serve to guide her future plans.

The answers to these questions will be quite different for students at varying stages in their education.

Regardless of where you are in your educational program, the career planning process involves thought, insight, and dedicated time. Although many resources are available for you to use in planning your career, the one most important to your career development is you! The career planning and development process is really about developing a life skill—one that you can apply not only in your educational and professional endeavours but also in your personal life.

THE DONNER-WHEELER CAREER PLANNING AND DEVELOPMENT MODEL

Career development is not a one-time activity, nor do you need to follow a step-by-step process. Once you have worked through the Model, you can move back and forth among the phases, adding and changing the content of your insights, information, and plans to reflect your developing career. The Model allows you to track your growth as a health care professional and to plan for your upcoming learning activities. In your educational program, you have built-in cues for when to "check in" with your career development. End of terms, evaluation times, and other program timelines or deadlines are transition times that you can use to guide and build on your work with the career model. The career development process will prompt you to do the following:

1. Understand and use the environment around you to develop your career.
2. Assess your growing strengths and development needs and validate that assessment.
3. Envision what your health-related career can be.
4. Develop a plan for using your educational activities in a way that will help you move toward your career vision.
5. Market yourself to achieve your career vision and related career goals.

Career development helps you stay focused and challenged so that you can create learning opportunities related to your goals or find meaning in experiences that, at face value, do not seem relevant or responsive to your immediate learning needs. The five phases of the Model include the items listed in the box below.

The Donner-Wheeler Career Planning and Development Model

Scanning Your Environment
What are the current realities and future trends?

Completing Your Self-Assessment
Who am I?
How do others see me?

Creating Your Career Vision
What do I really want to be doing?

Developing Your Strategic Career Plan
How can I achieve my career goals?

Marketing Yourself
How can I best market myself?

Planning Your Career

Y ou are now ready to learn to use the Donner-Wheeler Career Planning and Development Model (the Model). This chapter provides you with the details of each of the Model's five phases, along with examples from students' lives and experiences. The student examples are drawn from a number of health professions and are intended to illustrate how different phases of the Model can be used to help students shape their academic work. In each of the examples, the identified student program can be replaced by any health profession program—simply insert your program and take it from there! We have included activities to help you apply the Model to your particular educational level and personal and professional goals. Take time to review each phase carefully, and then proceed with the exercises. Remember, this is not a one-time activity but something you will want and need to come back to as you progress through your program and as your environment, experience, and interests change.

You can begin your work at any phase of the Model. Some health care professionals find it helpful to begin with scanning their environment to explore what is "out there" with a focus on (1) expanding their knowledge of the current issues and trends in health care and the career options within their profession, or (2) choosing a new direction in their career. Others choose to begin with their self-assessment as a strategy to reflect on, and articulate, their current strengths, areas for development, and recent accomplishments and follow this reflection with a scan of their environment with an eye to finding a fit between the outcome of their self-assessment and existing opportunities.

We have found that students find their initial work with the Model most exciting if they begin with creating their career vision. You begin with giving yourself the freedom to dream about what and who you wish to look like in the future.

CREATING YOUR CAREER VISION

What Is a Career Vision?

Your career vision describes where you want to go in your career and how you wish to fill your role as a health care professional; it is a description of you and what you wish to become. Your vision allows you to imagine what is possible and serves as a guide to how you can orchestrate your educational experiences to meet your career goals. Your vision can focus on who and what you wish to be in your career. Regardless of the focus, your vision provides you with a purpose and some insights into what you need to achieve your dream. Depending on the career options unique to your profession—and your own particular career interests—you may choose to create more than one career vision to guide and shape your academic activities.

Read through this section on creating your career vision; if you think you need to gather more information about your profession before you can create a meaningful vision, then go to the next section, "Scanning Your Environment." The scanning phase of the Model will help you scan the environment with a focus on understanding the current and emerging trends and issues in health care and in society generally and will enable you to consider various career options within your chosen profession. With this information, you can move on to creating your career vision.

Why Should You Have a Career Vision?

Having a career vision is perhaps the most forceful motivator for using all the components of your academic program and your summer and part-time work or volunteer opportunities to the fullest. Your vision can help you focus on how you can make the best of your learning opportunities rather than just reacting to events as they occur. Creating a career vision answers the question, "What do I want?" With an idea of what you would like your career to look like, you can approach any course and program experience with a sense of how it may help you get where you want to go. With each new encounter you have with the world of health care, your career vision may alter slightly or perhaps change altogether. Therefore, you should continually ask yourself, "Am I still feeling the way I felt about my profession when I entered my program? Does my career vision still reflect who and what I wish to be?" You can use a journal to continue to explore and reflect on this question as you move along in your program and your career. As a matter of fact, this would be a good time to begin keeping a journal of your thoughts and dreams. A journal is a powerful tool for keeping track of where you are headed and all the ideas and plans you have for getting there. It is your private record of who you are, what is important to you, and how you are changing. Many people have found a journal to be a valuable resource for "sorting things out."

Students are often uncertain about how they can design their career futures while still in their educational program. In most health profession programs, it is unlikely that individual students can choose their program requirements or select all their courses to suit their current interests. However, students can approach any classroom environment, field placement, or work or volunteer experience with focused goals that will help them progress toward their career vision. These personal learning goals may be an added dimension to the learning that is structured through the curriculum. Often, it is in academic experiences and opportunities that are seemingly unrelated to their career visions that students can be the most creative and active in shaping their learning. Many students find that when they optimize opportunities, as opposed to resisting the unknown, they end up discovering more choices than they had ever considered.

We suggest that you save your career vision in an electronic file. Print it, and place it where you can see it on a regular basis—most likely near your computer screen! Each time you sit down to contemplate an assignment or update your self-assessment, use your vision to guide your work and your focus. How can you best use your curricular activities to progress toward your vision? Be active in shaping your academic activities to ensure that they are helping you achieve your career vision. Keeping your vision close at hand also helps you recognize whether your vision is still what you wish it to be or if your recent experiences require that you either change it or further affirm that it remains true to your dream. As mentioned above, at any time in your academic career, you may have more than one career vision, or your vision may change as you gather diverse experiences and opportunities. Career visions are not written in stone; if elements of your vision change over time or you have a complete shift to a new vision, you can apply the Model to use what you have accomplished to create new opportunities and directions.

Carly created her career vision by using the questions outlined above as she began the third year of her social work program. Through the process of creating her vision, Carly realized that she had a dream for her career that she had not articulated, even to herself.

> I guess in the back of my mind I have always thought I would like to go to Africa and work in a community-based clinic. Walking through the questions to develop my vision, I realized that this is what I want to aim for and that I can start now to set myself up to actually do it. I feel an excitement and a sense of optimism about my future career that I have not felt for a while.

Carly developed an e-portfolio to keep track of her vision and other phases of the Model and included a picture of an African village to remind her why she was doing what she was doing and where she hoped to go. She printed both her written vision and the picture so that she could keep them in view when she worked at her computer.

VERONIKA Veronika a physiotherapy student, had a career vision that centred on her dream of being a physiotherapist in a neonatal follow-up clinic. Her field experience was in a long-term rehabilitation program, and she expressed concern that she would need to put her hopes for a neonatal focus "on hold" during this experience. In spite of a seeming lack of fit between her career vision as an expert in physiotherapy for children born prematurely and the area of long-term rehabilitation, she shared her vision with both her faculty advisor and a physiotherapist working in a long-term setting. She also met with her faculty mentor, who had expertise in pediatric physiotherapy. She was reminded by each of these resources that she could focus her learning goals on interpersonal and team communication skills as well as interdisciplinary practice. At the end of term, Veronika evaluated her rehabilitation experience as a most valuable learning experience in terms of refining her communication skills with both short-term and long-term clients and their families. She also discovered that the competencies she strengthened during this experience would serve her well when working with children and their families.

How to Create Your Own Career Vision

Creating a career vision involves *affirmation* (articulating a statement of what you want to create in your life), *visualization* (forming a picture or image of what you want to create), and *germination* (being committed to a vision you believe will be realized). It begins with taking time to do some active daydreaming about an ideal day in your future. Your career vision will be as individual as you are. To create it, you will need to ask yourself some important questions and give yourself permission to let go of what you previously thought possible.

Two general questions will guide you in this process. The questions, "What do I want?" and "What am I seeking?" will help you get started—rather like a warm-up or brainstorming session. No answer is wrong. The questions, "What is my ideal vision for my career?" and "What would my ideal day look like?" provide more focus as you begin to create your career vision. Formulate your career vision in the present tense as if it were occurring right now, and formulate it in as much descriptive detail as possible.

Olivia, a third-year nutrition student, created a career vision statement that reflected her progressive interest in being a member of a community health team:

> In one of my first-year nutrition courses, an alumna from my nutrition program who works in a community-based health centre spoke to the class about her role as a member of an interdisciplinary team in the centre. I didn't know that working in this type of centre would be an option for someone in my profession, and although I may not be able

ALI   Ali, an occupational therapy student, had just completed his final field placement of the year in a stroke recovery unit. He had the unexpected opportunity to work with a young adult and received feedback that he had made a positive difference in the rehabilitation experience of this patient's family.

Ali described his career vision as follows:

"I am an expert advanced occupational therapist, with particular expertise in working with young adults, practising in an active unit in a large teaching hospital located in a metropolitan city. I feel confident working with young adults and their families. I serve as a resource and clinical expert for my occupational health and interdisciplinary colleagues. I am seen by my colleagues as knowledgeable, approachable, and supportive with a high degree of professional integrity. The hospital in which I work supports my ongoing professional development and my practice. Clients and their families feel they can trust me to advocate for their needs. I leave each day feeling I have made a difference. When I arrive home, I have the energy to connect with my friends and family."

Although Ali was aware that his ultimate career vision might change as he encountered new areas of professional practice, he developed a vision that reflected his current hopes and dreams.

to gain employment in a community setting as a new graduate, my ultimate goal is to work in a health profession team caring for clients in a diverse community setting. I have created my career vision and am aware of how I can use course experiences to prepare to achieve my goals. I have also registered in the optional practicum course in my program to gain some experience in the field. On the advice of our director, I have joined our university mentorship program to develop communication and teaching skills that are important in my profession. Over the summer months, I plan to volunteer in our university health services clinic so that I can benefit from working with students in other professional programs with a focus on the university community. Finally, I have met a few times with the alumna who spoke to our class and have asked her to be my mentor. She has indicated that my curricular and volunteer experiences will hold me in good stead as I begin my career in the field of nutrition and believes that maintaining a focus on the competencies needed for community-centred practice can be achieved in any health-related setting. Although my vision changes slightly as I learn more about myself, my profession, and health care, the essence of my vision has remained fairly constant.

Olivia's Career Vision: I am an expert community-based nutrition expert with recognized expertise in the needs and care of individuals and communities. I work with an innovative interdisciplinary team that values the contributions of each team member. I am acknowledged as an informed team member with particular expertise in health teaching and promotion in the area of nutrition. I am responsive to the diverse needs of individuals and groups within the community. Together with my supportive colleagues, I know that I make a difference to the community at large. At the end of the day, I return home to my family with a sense of accomplishment and anticipation.

Your career vision can articulate the type of professional you wish to be or the particular area of your profession that is of most interest to you. For example, a first-year student in a speech-language pathology and audiology program developed the following career vision:

I am an expert speech-language pathologist who is recognized for my extensive knowledge base, my exceptional interpersonal skills, my practice excellence, and my commitment to collaborative school-based practice. My colleagues describe me as the person you want to have around when you are working—supportive, knowledgeable, kind, and accessible. I have fun at work and trust that my colleagues in both education and speech pathology share my commitment to working toward the highest quality of practice possible. I end my day knowing that I have done excellent work and am ready to enjoy an evening with my partner.

Lydia, a fourth-year student, created a career vision that reflected her desire to be an entrepreneur in her still undecided health service management practice specialty:

I am an independent health service management professional with specific research and practice expertise working in a consulting role. I work with individual clients and organizations to establish and evaluate programs in my area of health service management expertise. I am recognized for my knowledge, skill, and ability to work effectively and efficiently to produce a relevant "product" of excellent quality. I am known for my collaborative approach to projects and my commitment to ensuring that the work that we do makes a difference to the stakeholders. At the end of each day, I am confident that I have given my all to a project and have learned something new. I head to the gym and then home, where my dog and two cats are waiting for me!

Whether your career vision involves a specialty area within your particular health profession, a professional image, or both, it can serve as a motivating guide as you progress toward your dream.

Now you are ready to develop your career vision. Do Activity 1.

Activity Creating Your Career Vision

When you start, your vision does not need to be too realistic; that comes later in the process, when you set your career goals. Do not worry about your vision being too big, too vague, or too impossible. It should be grand and inspiring; if it is an important dream, it may even be a little scary.

Now, close your eyes, put your feet up, and picture yourself as a health care professional in your particular discipline doing exactly what you want to do, with whom you want to do it, and where you want to do it—and doing it well! Imagine yourself on a typical day, heading off to your ideal position in the workplace that allows you to do the best job possible. Use the following questions to guide your visioning exercise.

➢ Where do you live?

➢ What is the weather like as you head into work?

➢ How are you getting to work (e.g., walking, driving, cycling, or using public transit)?

➢ How do you feel as you head into your work day?

➢ What does the building in which you work look like? How does your workplace support you and your professional role?

➢ When you get to work, you overhear a colleague who knows you well describing you to an individual just starting her employment. What words does your colleague use to describe you?

➢ As you enter the area where your clients are, what kind of work will you be doing, and how do your clients perceive you?

➢ Who works most closely with you? How does your organization support your work?

➢ As you head home at the end of your day, how do you feel about what you have accomplished?

➢ What or who awaits you at the end of your day?

What Have You Accomplished?

You have a dream! This dream may change over the course of your educational program, or it may stay with you until your graduation. Either way, your dream can help you create and use your future learning activities. Your dream is your guide.

SCANNING YOUR ENVIRONMENT

What Is Scanning?

Scanning the environment involves simply looking around with the goal of identifying how your immediate and surrounding environment can help you work toward your career vision or, in some cases, create your vision. You have already been introduced to the process of scanning the environment as a student. Your curriculum helps you learn to plan your work with your client and to observe your client's environment and the variables that influence the client's well-being (e.g., resources, social factors, economic realities). Your program curriculum also offers you structured opportunities, usually in classes and seminars, to learn about important elements of an environmental scan, such as current issues in your profession, health care, work design, workplace options and foci (e.g., community, hospital, university, private practice, research, teaching), social determinants of health, and society at large. Each of these elements is important to consider within the context of your career vision.

Scanning the environment and then identifying your own strengths and interests will give you the information you need to identify possibilities for your current and future professional experiences, professional skill development, and course selection. Scanning helps you answer the following questions:

+ What opportunities are available in my profession that would help me progress toward my career vision?
+ What do I need to be aware of?
+ What and who are my resources?

The breadth of your environmental scan may vary depending on where you are in your program. In the early years of your program, you may find it most helpful to concentrate your scan on your school, curriculum requirements, field placement settings, and information available through these resources. As you begin your program, the primary focus of your scan is likely to be on discovering and using the school environment to your best advantage. As you advance, you will be looking toward preparing for graduation and entry to the profession. Your preparation will rely on a greater knowledge of what is happening outside your immediate learning environment. Extending your scan to include learning about health-related and profession-specific issues and trends locally, provincially, nationally, and even internationally will be an important next step.

As a student, you are at a definite advantage when doing an environmental scan. You have ready access to this information from your course work, from faculty members, and from any involvement you may have in field placements and volunteer activities. Using the scan to help you with your career planning is just another way to apply your learning. You are already ahead of the game!

Why Is Scanning Important?

Scanning helps you discover opportunities and resources within and outside your program, as well as current and future employment opportunities, by focusing on current and future trends in health care, your profession, and society as a whole. Your career vision reminds you of who and where you hope to be in the future. The process of scanning can help you make the best of your learning experiences and identify both short- and long-term goals and learning activities in keeping with your career vision. Without continuous scanning, it would be difficult to focus your development to your best advantage and to know the best direction in which to head and even more difficult to influence your learning activities and professional development.

How and When Do You Scan?

The simple answer is—continuously! You can scan throughout your educational program to learn what is happening now and what may happen in the future. Sources of information include the following:

✦ Course readings
✦ Discussions with faculty, preceptors, and mentors
✦ Professional and popular journals; printed and other forms of news media
✦ Internet
✦ Observations
✦ Friends and colleagues
✦ Everyday experiences
✦ Professional organizations
✦ Unions

Jordan, a nursing student, shares his belief that his professional organization is a great source of information:

> I find it very helpful to read clips from my professional organization. After joining as a student member, I was sent regular newsletters and media clips via e-mail. I find that these clips are really helpful in keeping me up to speed on what is happening locally, nationally, and globally in relation to my profession—and how I can make a difference, even as a student.

Reading, talking, and listening are the means you will use to make sense of the information you collect. As a student, you have the added benefit of a number of faculty members, professional resources, mentors, and student colleagues who are "at your fingertips" to help you direct, interpret, and use the information you will collect in your scan. Once you have gathered all the information, it is helpful to

SONJA Sonja, a third-year student, first used the environmental scan to look at an upcoming field placement with a focus on how this experience could help her develop the professional competencies required for her to achieve her vision of being a hospital-based physiotherapist working with clients who have experienced a sports-related injury and require rehabilitation. Sonja began her scan by obtaining a list of the course readings related to the upcoming program module addressing therapeutic exercise. A brief look at the readings gave her an idea of current issues and trends related to this module's focus, both nationally and locally. She then met a faculty member with expertise in sports-related rehabilitation physiotherapy. Their discussion about the nature of this rehabilitation physiotherapy and related roles within acute care settings helped her identify areas to focus on in her upcoming course and field experiences. Moreover, the faculty member was able to help Sonja develop some learning goals that could be achieved within her current placement that would also help her build the professional competencies needed for working effectively with clients with sports-related injuries. Her self-assessment would then help her identify her unique areas for development and specify learning objectives related to these competencies.

Recall Carly, the third-year student whose dream was to work in a community-based clinic in Africa. Carly used her vision to guide her environmental scan. She began her scan by checking her school Web site to find the research and practice interests of her program's faculty members. She discovered that a faculty member in her school of social work was involved in research related to sustainable social programs in Africa. Carly arranged a meeting with the faculty member, with whom she shared her vision of working in an African community. Her faculty contact was able to direct Carly to a colleague who worked at a teaching hospital nearby and who was leading an African mission with a focus on children and families with human immunodeficiency virus (HIV). From that contact, Carly was put in touch with two fourth-year students who had spent the previous summer doing volunteer health work in Africa. Her faculty contact also recommended elective courses that focused on both community development and interdisciplinary practice. Carly's scan was not a complex one; she focused on resources within her school of social work and ended up with a rich array of contacts and information on how she could best use her courses and field placements to develop competencies, in the short and long terms, that fit with her long-term vision. Her next step was to work on her self-assessment to determine how she could shape her learning experiences in the coming terms.

organize it into school, local, national, and global categories. You can add information to these categories at any time.

You should think of your scan as a work in progress, something you continually update and revise to reflect your growing experience, knowledge, and understanding of your chosen professional world. Students often complete a scan with the broad goal of determining how they can best shape their field placement experiences and course selection to advance toward their career vision. Hence, they may concentrate their scan on local and school-related trends, issues, and resources. Students in the latter years of their program find that extending their focus to provincial and national levels gives them the information they need to make decisions regarding what steps to take after graduation. The data from your scan can be guided by, and inform, your career vision. Whatever your vision and focus, try to make scanning an integral part of your everyday academic and personal lives.

Now that you understand what scanning is and how to use it, try Activity 2.

Activity (2) Scanning Your Environment

The trends and issues you identify in your scan can help you make decisions about potential opportunities within your classroom and external professional environments. Use your career vision to develop additional questions to guide your scan. What do you need to know to develop specific career goals and learning objectives that will help you capitalize on opportunities in your academic activities? The following are some general questions to ask.

➢ Is there someone who is the kind of health care professional I hope to be or currently doing the type of work I would like to do? What are the characteristics of that person or work?

➢ Are there environmental constraints I must consider when planning to do what I really want to do?

➢ What environmental supports or resources would facilitate my progress toward my career vision?

The following is a more detailed guide that can help you with your scan. Consider school, local, and national areas. If you feel ready to extend your scan to the global level, then include that category as well.

For each of the categories (school, local, national, global), consider issues related to society, health care in general, and your profession, within the context of your vision. Insert those trends and issues you observe to be important at this time as you consider where you are in your development and where you hope to be in the future. To help you fill in your scan, we have provided you with some questions to consider and a sampling of possible answers. Your list of questions and answers will likely grow over time.

Remember that you will need to review and revise your scan on a regular basis. The end of each term can be a cue to update your scan.

SCHOOL

➢ What are some of the opportunities or realities of your school setting?
Examples: components of the curriculum, required courses, program electives, extracurricular opportunities, faculty resources and mentors, student association representatives, interdisciplinary courses

LOCAL

➤ What are some of the important social and health issues in your local area?
Examples: changing demographics of the client population, a shift in health care to the community, interprofessional practice, poverty, access to care

➤ What are the important professional issues in your local area?
Examples: shortage or surplus of professionals in your discipline, changing professional practice settings, changing roles in the practice setting

NATIONAL

➤ What are the significant national health and social trends?
Examples: controlling health care costs, decreasing lengths of hospital stays, community-based care, increased use of technology, evidence-based practice, family-centred care

➤ What are the national issues affecting professionals in your discipline?
Examples: advanced entry to practice education, education specialization, quality of work life, funding, issues of health literacy

GLOBAL

➤ What health or social issues seem to be worldwide phenomena?
Examples: infectious diseases, ethical issues, allocation of resources, the gap between rich and poor people, social determinants of health

SCANNING YOUR ENVIRONMENT

School		
Curriculum/Courses	Field Placement Opportunities	Faculty Resources

Local Trends and Issues		
Society	Health Care	Profession

National Trends and Issues		
Society	Health Care	Profession

Global Trends and Issues		
Society	Health Care	Profession

What Have You Accomplished?

You have a vision for your career! Completing an initial environmental scan has given you some valuable information about what is available in your school, the issues professionals in your discipline currently face, and the type of opportunities available for your course and field experiences and how these opportunities can help you achieve your vision. This information helps you see what is possible and realistic so that you can make the best of your learning experiences.

What Is Your Next Step?

You now have a better understanding of your professional world and the health care world. The next step is getting a sense of how your interests, values, and abilities fit with your hopes for the future. This process is called self-assessment. After completing the self-assessment, you should do a reality check of it with others.

COMPLETING YOUR SELF-ASSESSMENT

What Is Self-Assessment?

Your self-assessment helps you identify your values, experiences, knowledge, strengths, and areas for development and then link them with your career vision and environmental scan to plan the next educational steps you wish to take. Your self-assessment helps you shift your vision from the future to the present. When you scanned the environment, you focused on noting what surrounds you and on building an understanding of how that influences your present and future development. The self-assessment focuses on you. It can assist you in recognizing all the attributes that make you who you are, what areas you would like to focus on for further development, and what you have to offer. Your self-assessment also provides you with the opportunity to think about how your personal life goals influence, and are influenced by, your career vision and choices.

Completing your self-assessment will allow you to give honest and accurate answers to the question, "Who am I?" When you put your self-assessment together with your vision and the results of your environmental scan, your replies will enable you to complete the last phases of the career planning and development process: developing your strategic career plan and marketing yourself to implement your plan.

Why Is Assessing Yourself Important?

As a student, an awareness of your values, skills, and strengths will provide insight into what you have brought to your profession and what areas you would like to develop further. It forms an important basis for making plans and developing the type of career and future that is congruent with your vision and is what you want.

Some students believe they have no say in planning their educational experiences. It is true that most health care curricula have required courses and learning activities, and you may not have a choice about taking those courses. However, you can choose how to interpret and use these courses to meet your unique needs. In addition to the required courses, there is usually a range of elective courses from which you can select according to your interests and preferences. Within both scenarios, your ability to use your learning to meet your professional and personal learning needs (which, preferably, are similar) depends on how well you know yourself. Self-knowledge of interests, values, knowledge, skills, strengths, and limitations can help you look at any experience as a meaningful learning opportunity. Sharing your assessment helps others respond to your unique needs.

In many ways, as a student, you have an advantage in this fundamental step of the career planning and development process. Most health profession curricula require that you participate in some form of self-reflection and self-evaluation. The key to success is to find meaning in the doing. Too often, students approach the process of self-evaluation and self-reflection as an academic exercise rather than as a means of enhancing their own career development. Once you claim the process of self-assessment as your own, you will be able to capitalize on your identified strengths and life experiences across all dimensions of your educational experiences. Revisiting your career vision and self-assessment at the end of each term will allow you to update your self-knowledge, set new learning goals, and develop career goals and action plans that will contribute to your ability to advance toward your vision. Using your self-assessment to guide your participation in your curriculum will give you the confidence to find or create meaning in your future learning experiences.

During or prior to your professional program, you may have used assessment tools such as the Myers-Briggs Type Inventory (a personality test), the Leadership 360 Assessment (an assessment that includes feedback from a number of sources, including fellow employees, supervisors, and others), and more general learning style inventories. If you have used these or other assessment tools, you may find such previous work helpful as you move forward on this phase of the Model.

Beginning the Self-Assessment Process

The first questions are "Who am I?" and "How would I describe myself?" Answering these questions involves much more than describing what you do or where you are in your educational preparation. Even though you spend a considerable amount of time at school (and perhaps at work) to support your academic endeavours, it is important to acknowledge those other components that complete your life, including your personal health, well-being, and development; your family and friends; your community; and your personal life goals.

Although you may be new to your chosen health care profession, you have had valuable life experiences prior to entering your program that have contributed to your current professional strengths. For example, think about all the adjectives you could use to describe what makes you unique. Although we are all unique, the challenge lies in being able to articulate that uniqueness. Can you make a list of three characteristics that define your uniqueness? Think back to your visioning experience. Often the adjectives you envisioned your colleagues using to describe you reflect your current unique attributes. Pick up a pencil and paper and make that list—now! Keep that list, and refer to it and revise it from time to time. Who we are includes our beliefs and values, our knowledge and skills, our interests, and our hopes for our futures. *Beliefs* are the way in which we view ourselves and the world around us. *Values* are a set of beliefs that drive our decisions, actions, reactions, behaviours, and relations. *Knowledge and skills* are the abilities and behaviours we use to produce results, and *interests* are the activities on which we like to spend most of our time and from which we gain pleasure.

Assessing Your Values

Values are those principles we prize and cherish—those beliefs we hold as extremely important. Values direct our decisions and influence our lives. As you begin to identify your values, consider why you chose your particular profession as a career and how your experiences to date fit with those values. Ask yourself the following questions:

✦ What is important to me in my educational and personal lives?
✦ What significant experiences or interests prompted me to consider my profession as a career?
✦ Who has inspired me in my professional education, and what values did that person convey to me?
✦ What can I contribute to my profession?
✦ What values influence my professional learning and overall development?
✦ Who or what are the significant people or things in my life that I need to consider at this time?
✦ What are my priorities—self, partner, family, school, work, community, or other?

Read your career vision and identify the values that are embedded in that vision. Those values may relate to what you need to have in your workplace to be satisfied (e.g., support for ongoing learning, resources that allow you to offer a high quality of care, colleagues who share your commitment to quality care). Your vision may also highlight values related to your ability to make a difference, remain passionate about what you do, have fun, and experience a sense of collegiality. Your hopes for the future can offer you insight into what you value as an individual in your profession.

If you find that you are having difficulty articulating your values, there are many resources that can help you with values clarification. The "Career Planning and Development Resources" section in this guide includes two online sources related to values clarification that may help you as you work on this important phase of your career planning and development.

MARILYN Marilyn recognized the strong influence her father had on her choice to become a pharmacist. Her father, who had been a pharmacist, exemplified professionalism, knowledge, caring, and strength—the qualities Marilyn associated with the role of a pharmacist. In addition to demonstrating respect for the uniqueness and integrity of each individual, Marilyn's father was an excellent educator, both with clients and with the people with whom he worked. He was also someone who saw change as an opportunity to learn and to increase the quality of service and care he offered to clients. For example, when technology was introduced in pharmacy, Marilyn's father embraced it with enthusiasm and integrated it into his practice such that it allowed him and his colleagues to offer comprehensive health education and direct service to a diverse client group.

Marilyn also had the opportunity to observe her father's interaction with clients of all ages and witnessed the positive effect her father had on his clients through his professional presence and individualized approach. Marilyn developed an interest in pharmacy as a career, with a vision of working in a community-based pharmacy located in an area with diverse clients. In addition, her teachers, family members, and friends told her she was very good with people and would make a great pharmacist. Her vision of being a warm, caring, and committed professional interested in working closely with clients of all ages and backgrounds helped Marilyn to articulate her values and to keep these in mind as she evaluated various field experiences and academic activities.

Marilyn states, "It's funny. I think that I knew from an early age that I wanted to be a pharmacist, but it wasn't until I sat down and really thought about why I wanted to be a pharmacist that I realized what an excellent role model my father has been and how that modelling has influenced my decision to go into pharmacy, with a vision toward a community-based pharmacist role. I can see how I have come to value many of the things my father does and how these values will help me be a reputable pharmacist."

Assessing Your Knowledge and Skills

Career visions provide information about the breadth and depth of the professional competencies you will require to actualize your hopes for the future. The self-assessment process allows you to consider where you are at now relative to where you are going.

Recognizing what knowledge and skills you possess—and to what degree you possess them—is a crucial outcome of the self-assessment process. Knowledge develops through a combination of formal learning and experience, whereas skills are acquired abilities. By reviewing your past accomplishments, field and classroom evaluations, volunteer activities, and program goals, you can begin to identify your strengths and the areas you would like to develop further. Consider your career vision and the work you have done in your professional program and in your nonprofessional life. Your community and social environments also provide opportunities for acknowledging your current strengths and increasing your knowledge and skills with regard to people and the world in which you live.

As you accumulate experiences in your academic program, you will gather feedback related to your strengths, your progress, and areas to develop from a variety of instructors, peers, and professional practice contacts. Share your vision with those who you think can help you assess your current strengths and who can assist you in targeting areas for development. In the past, job requirements tended to relate only to job duties and not to work attitudes, general communication, and interpersonal skills. When you sit down to evaluate your professional competencies, take into account your personality and nature, your attitude, the way you work with others, and the ease with which you communicate. These attributes are highly transferable and highly valued by health care organizations.

Recognizing limitations or gaps in your knowledge and skills is just as important as acknowledging your strengths. If you do not recognize these limitations, you may miss important learning opportunities.

You should ask yourself the following questions:

+ What knowledge and skills did I bring with me when I entered my program?
+ What knowledge and skills have I developed, both personally and professionally?
+ What are my strengths?
+ What are my limitations?
+ What knowledge and skills require further development?

Many of the successes and strengths you have enjoyed in other areas of your life will hold you in good stead in your health care career. If you are in the first year of your program, start by considering your past accomplishments, focusing on the values, insight, skills, and strengths that you developed as a result of your efforts.

ELLIOTT Elliott's career vision focused on working as a respiratory therapist in a neonatal intensive care transport team. He wished to be considered a valued, knowledgeable, resourceful, and committed member of the transport team.

Elliott identified his involvement on his high school rowing team as an accomplishment. When he focused on the skills he had developed as a result of this experience, he identified strengths in teamwork, an ability to successfully balance academic and extracurricular activities, and skill in coaching new team members effectively. Reflecting on his positive experiences with his rowing team also helped Elliott realize how much he valued working as part of a team. Each of these skills and insights would be an asset to him as he participated in his academic career with an eye to his vision.

SIARA Siara's career vision placed her in the role of an expert pharmacist at an active teaching hospital. She saw herself involved in working at an interdisciplinary level to manage and create systems to ensure that patients frequently on complex medication regimens received safe and effective therapy. Siara would like to teach health profession students in the hospital setting about pharmaceutical care. She would also like to be involved in research studies on pharmaceutical care and patient safety, with a particular focus on the field of oncology.

During high school, Siara was a volunteer counsellor for three summers at a camp for children with cancer. She worked closely with the counselling team to ensure that the children were provided with a safe environment. She was struck by the amount of medication that each child required as part of their health care. She had many discussions with the camp nurse, who explained the different medications. The nurse also spoke highly of the pharmacist who had established the medication delivery system for the children and had provided information about the medications, their effects, and potential interactions and complications both to the nurse and to the counsellors who were not health care professionals. By the end of her final summer at the camp, Siara had learned a great deal about medications frequently used in the treatment of cancer in children and how different medications affected each child's physical and emotional well-being. She was able to identify her awareness of the importance of an interdisciplinary approach in health care and was acknowledged for her strengths in teamwork, initiative, responsibility, and compassion.

After identifying your strengths and skills, focus on enhancing them in the context of your professional experience by asking for specific feedback and by seeking experiences that meet your unique learning needs. Being aware of your values can also add insight and clarity to your reflection and evaluation of each learning experience. Use the journaling process to reflect on the impact of your experiences on your evolving professional competencies, and your career vision can foster a sense of focus and progress.

Assessing Your Interests

Interests provide another guide to determine your current and future learning goals and to decide how you would ideally like to meet those goals. They can be grouped into four categories:

+ People: helping, serving, caring for, or selling things to people
+ Data: working with facts, records, or files
+ Things: working with machines, tools, or living things such as plants and animals
+ Ideas: creating insights, theories, or new ways of saying or doing something

What have you liked about your past and current jobs, summer employment, part-time jobs, academic jobs (e.g., research assistant, work-study student), or volunteer activities? What did you dislike? In what type of environment do you learn and perform at your best? What do you like to do outside of the academic environment or your current workplace? What energizes or motivates you? Answering these questions will help you understand and articulate your interests.

Recognizing Your Accomplishments

Accomplishments are those specific successes that have marked the highlights of your performance in any of your roles (e.g., as student, volunteer, or employee). For example, you may have developed a client teaching package, provided an in-service for the staff at your field placement, or received acknowledgement or recognition for your strong communication or leadership skills in your student role. These accomplishments represent those times in your life when you made a difference. They become the added value that you will bring to any health care environment.

Data from your career vision, environmental scan, and self-assessment help you interpret and structure your learning experiences in a way that is relevant and meaningful to you. The more you learn and reflect on your development as a health care professional, the more you can begin to influence your learning experiences.

JAKE Jake was in the process of planning for his upcoming field placement in the community. His career vision focused on the kind of professional he wished to be. He admired occupational therapists (OTs) who could focus well on the people with whom they worked—clients, families, and colleagues. He also strove to emulate OTs who could establish positive and meaningful relationships while demonstrating exceptional knowledge of occupational therapy practice. A detailed self-assessment was invaluable to Jake. While completing his self-assessment, he discovered that he (1) valued the continuity of working with older adults; (2) was interested in working with people over time, particularly in home intervention; (3) needed a greater knowledge of the health care resources that were available in the community for the older adult living at home; and (4) needed further development in the area of interprofessional approaches to the care of the older adult. Jake created a career plan to guide his approach to his upcoming field placement. His plan acknowledged his existing strengths and focused on those competencies needed to effectively assess and manage the care of clients requiring home intervention. Through his environmental scan, Jake had identified general trends in occupational therapy practice in long-term home care. On the basis of information from his scan and self-assessment, he decided to request a focus on community home care programs targeting older adults who were in need of occupational therapy in their homes. If this request could not be accommodated, Jake asked that he have a field placement that would afford him the opportunity to advance his knowledge of community health care resources and interdisciplinary practice.

In most health profession educational programs that have field placement as a component or opportunity in the curriculum, students are required to complete these field placements in organizations that provide experiences congruent with the general goals of the curriculum. Knowing the competencies necessary to achieve expertise in your area of interest can help you make the best of any practice experience, even if the particular placement is not of your choosing. Your career vision, together with a comprehensive scan of the environment and data from your self-assessment, will provide you with the information you need to capitalize on available learning opportunities.

In the previous example, Jake's awareness of his values, interests, knowledge, and areas for further development provided a direction for his professional educational goals that he could use to guide his learning in any setting. By formulating a learning plan focused on (1) skill development for the care of clients in a community setting, (2) interdisciplinary practice, and (3) his particular interest in the older adult client, he could shape his practice learning experience to enhance his skills in working with older adults needing occupational health care in a community context.

Another senior-level student described how information from the self-assessment process helped him evaluate different learning experiences:

> Throughout my 4 years, I would imagine "putting on the hat" of a specialty of my profession that had caught my attention, and I would create a career vision for each "hat." I would gather information about this particular area through reading, talking to professionals working in the area, and attending conferences. I was assessing the match between my interests and talents (gathered through the self-assessment) and the specialty that interested me at that time.

Through ongoing self-assessment, this student recognized his strength in interpersonal communication, specifically in the establishment of therapeutic goal-directed relationships with individual clients. This self-knowledge helped him evaluate the fit between an area of professional practice and a unique professional skill:

> I became interested in informatics and had a related career vision. I went to conferences, read books, and talked to some professionals in the informatics area. I imagined the work I would be doing and explored what I would need to get involved. In the end, it didn't feel right to me. I liked computers and had a good idea of their potential in health care, but I wanted to work more with people and ideas, not with machines, data, and policy. My interest in informatics as a career focus faded and was replaced by a new interest—a new "hat"—and a vision that was more congruent with my values and strengths.

A third-year student found that by keeping her values at the centre of her professional work, she was able to develop competencies and expertise that would be an asset in any setting:

> My aunt has a disability and has worked tirelessly to advocate for the right of disabled individuals to participate fully in society. I chose a disability studies program to learn to do what she does—to take informed risks, to advocate for myself and others, and to make a difference. I am not sure where I want to focus my work, but my vision is that I am known for my expertise in advocacy, lobbying, and proactive political action and that I am perceived as caring and just. Knowing this, I make it a point to make the development of competencies related to these attributes a career focus in each of my academic experiences.

Now you are ready to complete your self-assessment in Activity 3.

Activity (3) Completing Your Self-Assessment

With your vision and your environmental scan in mind, consider the following questions. They can help you understand who you are and what is important to you. Your answers will give you the words to describe your unique self, what you like to do, and what you have to offer. As you document your answers, you can begin to write your own story. Your story should include all of the important personal and professional events in your life and how they relate to one another.

1. VALUES: WHAT ARE MY PRIORITIES?

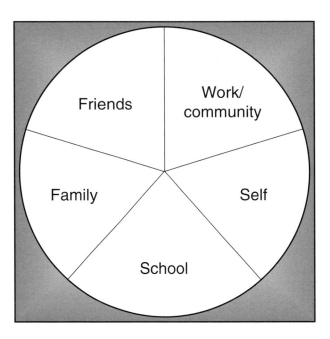

Mark the percentage of time you spend daily in each section of the circle. Now ask yourself the following questions.

➢ What is most important to me in my current educational experiences?
Examples: access to professional role models, opportunity to spend time with clients, program responsiveness to current health care realities, respectful relationships with teachers and student colleagues, acceptance of differences, accessible and approachable faculty members

➢ What is important to me as a student and in my personal life?
Examples: relationships, fairness, honesty, balance, social justice, knowing my strengths and limitations

➢ What are my key values?

➢ Who or what are the significant persons or things in my life that I need to consider at this time?
Examples: spending time with family, spouse or partner, boyfriend or girlfriend; part-time job; involvement in my community; volunteer activities

2. KNOWLEDGE AND SKILLS

➢ What knowledge and skills have I developed both personally and professionally in my program and outside of my educational experiences?
Examples: self-directed learning, resourcefulness, flexibility, organization, activism, effective teamwork

➢ What new knowledge and skills have I acquired since my last self-assessment?
Examples: assessment and evaluation skills, leadership skills, therapeutic communication skills, health teaching skills

➢ What are my strengths?
Examples: communication skills [specifically empathy, open-ended questions, and establishing positive rapport]; organizational skills; responsibility and accountability; resourcefulness, eagerness, and enthusiasm

➢ What are my areas for focused professional development?
Examples: active contribution to interprofessional teams, skills in advocacy, work with diverse clients and colleagues, conflict resolution

➢ What knowledge and skills would I like to develop in my current or next term?
Examples: theory related to advocacy, family-centred care theory in a community care context, effective client teaching, legal and ethical issues related to outpatient care

➢ What is my preferred learning style?
Examples: visual, auditory, tactile, kinesthetic, verbal
(If you are not aware of various learning styles, you can simply search Google, using the term "learning styles," for an introduction to the various types of learning styles. With this information, you can further explore the literature related to learning styles should you require further guidance in describing your values.)

3. INTERESTS

➢ What were my interests before I entered my program?

➢ What have I liked about my field experiences?
Examples: developing therapeutic relationships with clients, professional role modelling, positive teamwork

➤ What program-related experience has been most exciting for me, and why?
Examples: rehabilitation in which I was able to spend time getting to know clients; a slower pace in which I felt I had more control and independence in how I organized my care; time to consult and collaborate with other health care professionals

➤ What courses have been of most interest to me?

➤ What program experiences or courses have I disliked?
Example: I liked them all because I learned something in each one. The ones that were fast paced and "technical" were not as rewarding to me although I learned a lot about organization.

➤ What energizes or motivates me?
Examples: receiving positive feedback from faculty; hearing—from clients—that I do make a difference; meeting my own goals; relaxing with family and friends; having a good workout

➤ In what type of learning environment (class, field, extracurricular) do I perform my best?
Example: any environment in which there is interaction and a lot of discussion and in which I feel that what I have to say or contribute is important

➤ What do I like to do outside of my academic environment?
Examples: spend time outdoors, read, spend time with the people I care about, exercise

➤ What is important to me in my physical environment?
Examples: being located in a warm climate, being located in a rural or urban setting, being located close to my friends and family, being located away from familiar places and people

4. ACCOMPLISHMENTS

➤ What have been my most significant accomplishments in my professional education to date? Outside of my education?
Examples: elected as student representative on school council; told by my employer that I was an excellent "trainer" for new staff; told by my faculty that I have very good leadership skills for my level; have a lot of good friends and am a good friend to others

➤ Can I describe those times in my life when I made a difference?
Examples: When I had my placement at the rehabilitation unit, I organized a game show for the residents and staff. The staff said they had not seen the residents have so much fun in a long time.

Your Reality Check

The final part of self-assessment, the reality check, is about seeking feedback regarding your strengths and key areas for development. The reality check can help you broaden your view of yourself because others often see you differently from the way you see yourself. Once you have crafted your career vision, conducted your environmental scan, and answered the question, "Who am I?" it is important to validate your answers by doing a reality check. It will provide information that will help you answer the next critical question, "How do others see me?"

Students often find that the reality check provides an opportunity to be informed or reminded of strengths and attributes that they do not recognize in themselves. Keep in mind that your social, family, and community networks are also important sources of feedback about your knowledge, skills, strengths, and limitations. Armed with your vision and with regular formal evaluations from faculty, peers, and professional contacts, as well as with your expanding experience and your initial assessment of your accomplishments as you enter your profession, you can update your self-assessment on an ongoing basis.

Why Is a Reality Check Crucial?

Feedback affirms where we shine and sometimes identifies knowledge or skill gaps that need to be filled. As a student, you receive and respond to feedback on a continual basis. A good deal of the feedback you receive is tied to specific course or curriculum goals. Although this feedback is of value in determining and reinforcing your expanding professional strengths and areas for further development, it may not address the areas of self-assessment that you would like confirmed or viewed from another perspective. Therefore, be prepared to request specific feedback related to your self-assessment if your course and program feedback does not address all your unique needs.

How Do You Do a Reality Check?

Start with those individuals you trust—family, student peers, your mentor, and others who know you well. Then consider getting feedback from an individual whom you do not know too well (perhaps a preceptor or another health care professional) and ask him or her the same questions. You can also refer to your field placement evaluations and course feedback. The reality check component of the self-assessment process can strengthen your confidence in communicating your skills and uniqueness to colleagues, potential employers, and other professionals. For example, during the reality check step, a third-year social work student became aware of a strength she had not previously identified:

> I took my career vision and self-assessment to a faculty member whom I really like and respect. She confirmed the strengths that I had identified and, to my surprise, added something that I never would have considered. She said my sense of humour was excellent and that it allowed me to establish rapport with clients in a very gentle and non-threatening manner. Now when I work with clients, I am conscious of my use of humour and can see that it is unique and can be therapeutic. She also connected me with others who do the kind of work that I hope to do in the future.

Now you are ready to do your reality check. Complete Activity 4.

Activity (4) Reality Check

> **R**eview your career vision and self-assessment and re-read your accomplishments. Then, ask yourself the questions listed below.

➤ What feedback have I received from faculty members, preceptors, mentors, clients, student colleagues, friends, and family regarding my achievements?

➤ What did they identify as my strengths and key areas for development?

➤ What three adjectives would they (or did they) use to describe me, both within and outside the academic or professional practice environment or workplace? Why?

➤ How did my assessment of my accomplishments compare with others' assessments?

➤ What has changed since my last reality check?

Piece together all the data, and create a written summary of your strengths and challenges. With an accurate sense of who you are and how others see you, you will be ready to explore a range of opportunities and determine how you can focus your next learning experience.

What Have You Accomplished?

You have put your dream into words. The environmental scan gave you valuable information to consider and use to understand issues, trends, and resources, focusing on your career vision and on your chosen profession at several levels. Your self-assessment has allowed you to think about what is important to you, what you do well, and what you need to learn and develop further so that you can progress toward your career vision. Together, your vision, scan, and self-assessment help you get a sense of the fit and gaps between where you are now and where you wish to be in the future.

What Is Your Next Step?

Action! The next step of the career planning process guides you in making plans to use your educational program to determine what you need to learn to move toward your career vision. You know what is around you, you know yourself, and you have your dream. Go for it!

DEVELOPING YOUR STRATEGIC CAREER PLAN

What Is a Career Plan?

A career plan is like the learning plans you may be asked to develop throughout your academic career. In fact, as you advance in your education, your learning plan should be your career plan. Whether you view your learning plan and your career plan as one plan or as two separate plans, your career plan will guide you in working with your educational supports and resources to achieve your career goals.

A strategic career plan is a blueprint for action. You are now ready to specify the goals, activities, timelines, and resources you need to achieve your career vision. In this part of the process, you start to put on paper the specific strategies you will use to take charge of your future. The strategic career plan is always a work-in-progress, the object of continual evaluation. As a student, you will be constantly revisiting your vision, scanning your environment, assessing yourself, receiving feedback from others, and evaluating and re-evaluating your goals and your plans for reaching them.

Why Should You Develop a Career Plan?

Having a strategic plan helps you take advantage of each planned or unanticipated learning experience. Whatever your career vision and specific career goals, a plan will allow you to recognize unexpected or "accidental" learning experiences as opportunities and, ultimately, to take control of a rewarding career.

The key to a good plan is to ensure that it is both uniquely yours and easily converted into action within your educational experience. It must be derived from your career vision and outline specific actions that you can take to achieve clearly defined goals. Having a strategic career plan helps you make the career goals that are related to your career vision action oriented. You may have more than one strategic career plan at the same time, as stated by one student:

> In such turbulent times, I feel that I must have several backup plans ready to go at once. I keep my career vision true to my values and interests but fairly broad because I must be ready to shift my specific career goals or options at the drop of a hat. This flexibility and multiple career options allow me to sleep at night, knowing that if I don't get a particular job, I have lots of other possibilities that are still in keeping with my career vision.

How Should You Plan?

A strategic career plan includes identification of the following:

+ Goals
+ Action steps
+ Resources
+ Timelines
+ Indicators of success

Document your plan—in writing. The exercise of "writing it down" forces you to include each of the critical components and makes it easier for you to continually review, refine, evaluate, and re-evaluate both your goals and your progress. It also helps you make a commitment to yourself to work on making your plan become reality.

Set Goals

With your career vision, environmental scan, and self-assessment completed, set your short-term and long-term career goals, or your vision will remain only a dream. Choosing and setting goals means that you are serious about taking charge of your learning. When choosing your career goals, always ask yourself, "What do I hope to achieve by pursuing this goal?" Remember to keep the goals specific, time framed, reachable, and relevant. Will anyone who reads them understand what you are trying to accomplish? Do you have actual target dates for achievement? Are your goals realistic enough to be attainable? Are the goals in tune with your future needs?

Career goals should be realistic (I can do it), desirable (I want to do it), and motivating (I will work to make it happen). Remember that you will re-evaluate and alter your career goals as you move toward your career vision, or you may perhaps change your vision as you encounter new experiences in your educational program. Even if you change your vision, you can build on the activities and resources you have used in meeting previous goals.

MIYU To begin a strategic career plan, Miyu, a third-year student with a career vision of being a registered dietitian in a renal transplantation unit, developed the following goals:

Career Vision: I am an expert registered dietitian (RD) in an active transplant unit in a large urban teaching hospital. I work with an interdisciplinary team to provide a high quality of family-centred care to adults who have undergone kidney transplantation and to their families. I feel confident in my role as an RD within a highly collaborative interprofessional team dedicated to the care of clients following kidney transplantation. I am perceived by my colleagues to have expertise in family-centred care. I serve as a preceptor to students who have been selected to complete an internship in the area in which I work. My contributions are valued, and in return, I demonstrate my respect for the contributions of others. My organization supports both formal and informal professional development philosophically and financially. I enjoy going to work each day.

(Miyu is aware that to be eligible to write the RD college examination, she needs to complete a 1-year internship, likely in a teaching hospital, after obtaining her 4-year degree. The internships are highly competitive, so it is important that she make the best of her program so that she can be in the best position to secure an internship. The internship application process will likely require that Miyu submit a résumé and be interviewed. Miyu will need to develop a professional résumé and practise effective interviewing skills.)

Career Goal for the Academic Year: At the end of the fourth year of my nutrition program, I will have the necessary professional competencies to be considered for a dietitian internship position in an acute care environment where I can advance those competencies necessary to achieve my vision.

Short-Term Goals:

1. Use academic experiences, including a practicum course and courses required to write the RD examination, to develop competencies that will position me for an internship position in an acute care setting.
2. Connect with program alumni who were successful in obtaining an internship.
3. Find a mentor in the School of Nutrition with expertise in my area of interest.
4. Network with renal transplantation unit RDs through the professional organization and contacts provided by my mentor and school faculty members.
5. Develop a résumé that reflects my academic and extracurricular accomplishments and activities relevant to the internship, related professional competencies, and the organization offering the internship.
6. Feel confident about being interviewed.
7. Obtain a summer job in food services in a health care institution.

Long-Term Goal: Work as an RD in a renal transplantation unit.

Specify Action Steps

Once you have determined your goals, use specific action steps to further break down goals into discrete and concrete activities. Action steps complete the sentence, "In order to achieve this goal, I will . . . ."

MIYU Miyu chose the following action steps to achieve her short-term goals:

1. Through my environmental scan, identify the overall professional skills and specific professional competencies that are most important for acceptance into an internship program.
2. Update my self-assessment with these competencies in mind.
3. Meet with the program director to discuss potential curricular and extracurricular experiences that may help me develop those competencies identified in my self-assessment.
4. Talk to up to three faculty members who could possibly be mentors helping me to achieve my vision.
5. Find the names of program alumni who have had internships in an acute care environment and (if at all possible) who work in a transplantation unit in order to discuss the internship experience.
6. Develop my "junk drawer" résumé (see page 59) that includes all of my professional experiences (with a brief description of the skills and accomplishments resulting from each experience), professional and nonprofessional jobs, volunteer activities, extracurricular professional development activities, and professionally related qualifications.
7. Practise interviewing skills.
8. Check job postings for summer employment in the area of food services, particularly in health-related settings.

Identify Resources

Having identified specific action steps to take, you are now ready to look at the resources you may need to achieve your goal. The process of developing a plan requires you to think about who and what will help you implement your plan. Making a thoughtful inventory of your available and potential resources is the first step you should take to begin to implement the action steps associated with each of your goals.

> **MIYU** To achieve her goals, Miyu identified as resources (1) the student association representative in her school, (2) her program director, (3) program alumni, (4) a potential mentor, (5) the career centre at her school, and (6) local hospital employment postings in food services.

Once you have determined the resources you will require, you will be ready to set timelines to accomplish your action steps.

Establish Timelines

If your goal is personally motivating and your plan is realistic and concrete, assigning timelines ensures that you allocate your resources in an efficient and ultimately rewarding way. Timelines should be suited to your particular needs and fit your personal priorities. In the previous example, Miyu realized she would need to achieve most of her action plans by the due date for applications for internships. She gave herself 5 weeks to achieve all of her action plans, and she scheduled one to two specific action steps per week.

Timelines can be modified, but including them at the outset is critical to developing an effective career plan.

Identify Indicators of Success

How will you know that your plan is working? If you have documented your plan (including specific action steps, required resources, and timelines), you have a good start at identifying indicators of success. Think about what you are hoping to accomplish with your plan. For Miyu, identifying the indicators of success involved creating a list of professional competencies needed to be considered for an internship position; revising her self-assessment; and meeting with the program director, program alumni, the student association representative, and (hopefully) a mentor.

As you design your own plan, think about what success would look like for you. Career plans should be dynamic, responsive to personal circumstances, and professionally stimulating. You should be ready to adjust your plan as aspects of your vision or self-assessment change, as your continually updated environmental scan indicates that significant changes have occurred around you, and as you move forward in your education.

Now you are ready to develop your own strategic career plan. Complete Activity 5.

Activity (5) Developing Your Strategic Career Plan

> **A** well-developed strategic plan not only helps you realize your career vision but also enables you to recognize and take advantage of other career opportunities as they occur. Develop your strategic career plan by doing the following:
> + Start by placing your written career vision right in front of you.
> + Identify your short-term and long-term career goals.
> + Complete the strategic career plan outline shown below.

STRATEGIC CAREER PLAN OUTLINE

Career Vision:

Career Goals:

Action Steps	Resources	When to Accomplish	How Will I Know I Have Succeeded?

Thinking of Graduate Studies?

Pursuing graduate studies may have been your intent from the beginning of your education, or it may be a more recent decision arising from your career vision.

As with any other career decision, you have some important choices to make. Many students ask the following questions:

- ✦ How do I choose the right graduate program?
- ✦ How do I compare the benefits of one program or university with those of another?
- ✦ What types of questions should I be asking?
- ✦ What can I be doing in my undergraduate program to position myself for success in both application process and program of study?

You can use your strategic career plan to answer these important questions. You can integrate the career plan specific to your graduate studies into your existing career planning work (i.e., into every phase), or you might actually do a parallel career planning exercise devoted specifically to the pursuit of graduate studies. Either way, you can begin by expanding your environmental scan to include the nature and role of graduate programs in your profession or in related disciplines. Gather information about the types of available programs and how they advance the careers of health care professionals in your area of interest. You can also learn about general graduate education entry requirements (i.e., those that are usually required regardless of the university or program). With the information from your scan in mind, return to your self-assessment and focus on identifying gaps and strengths most relevant to this career planning strategy. For example, because grades and grade point average or class standing are almost always a key issue in graduate applications, review your grades, and (if necessary) consider how you can ensure that you meet the general requirements.

The next step in the development of your strategic career plan for graduate studies can focus on gathering information about the types of programs offered, the mode of delivery (online, campus based, or a mix or hybrid of online and campus-based modes), faculty resources, flexibility of programs with respect to full-time and part-time study options, access to online courses, timelines for degree completion, and career opportunities during and on completion of the program. Remember to ask for the philosophy and mission statement of the program so that you can determine whether the stated values and beliefs about teaching and learning are a good fit with the values you have identified in your self-assessment. Reviewing the profiles of faculty members at the schools of interest is another way to see whether the program has a faculty with expertise in your fields of interest. You can also arrange to meet with resource persons within the faculty and with alumni or current students in the program to discuss your questions. Do not forget that with each contact you are marketing yourself at the same time you are seeking information. The next section of this guide "Marketing Yourself" (concerning the fifth phase of the Model) offers specific marketing tips and strategies.

Use your self-knowledge and your career vision to assess congruency among your values, interests, learning style, career goals, and the various graduate programs. You can then more accurately assess how well any program will help you progress toward your career vision. This is where knowing the theoretical biases and approaches to teaching and learning, among other program characteristics, can help you make a decision that is a good fit with who you are, how you learn, and what is important to you. At any stage of this process, it can be helpful to seek the perspective of your mentor, student colleagues, and significant others. It can also be beneficial to speak with students you know who are currently engaged in a graduate program or who are recent graduates. Informal sources of information and guidance are often valuable resources as you prepare for your graduate education.

As you can see, using your strategic career plan to prepare for graduate studies prompts you to revisit all stages of the Model with a specific focus in mind. The work you will do as you explore graduate studies illustrates the dynamic nature of the career planning and development process and how it guides you in your efforts to achieve your career dreams.

What Have You Accomplished?

You have a game plan! You have used your vision, your environmental scan, and your self-assessment to develop some plans that you can begin to implement now. You have a concrete place to start. Your vision is on its way to becoming a reality.

What Is Your Next Step?

It is time to start telling others what you have just confirmed for yourself. You have a vision; you know your current strengths, values, interests, and accomplishments; you know how they fit with the world of health care; and you have a plan. Now you need to share all of this with the people who can help you.

MARKETING YOURSELF

Health Profession Students as Self-Marketers

Marketing simply means being able to communicate confidently and effectively to others your vision, strengths, interests, and goals, as well as the contributions you can make to professional practice. What better place is there than your education to acquire self-marketing skills?

A third-year student made the following comments about self-marketing:

> Although I was already aware of the importance of developing a career plan, I learned that the process does not end there; rather, the plan needs to be put into action through the use of various self-marketing strategies. I want to make sure I get the job that is right for me. For this reason, I feel it is important to implement appropriate self-marketing strategies so I can represent myself in the best possible way.

The key to successful marketing is to develop an approach that is congruent with your values and communication style and true to your abilities. When you completed your self-assessment, you identified your values and beliefs and evaluated your expanding professional experience, accomplishments, strengths, and areas for improvement. Now that you have taken a close look at the things that make you unique, you can most effectively promote yourself and meet your goals by making and keeping yourself visible. Your strengths, coupled with a commitment and a belief in yourself, make you your own best marketer.

Why Marketing Yourself Is Important

Intentionally or unintentionally, you market who and what you are in every professional encounter. During each field placement experience, each involvement in the classroom environment, and each meeting with a faculty member or student colleague, you communicate (directly or indirectly) your values and your professional identity. Thoughtful and intentional self-marketing enables you to take control of how you represent yourself to others. In this section, you will learn about the resources and tools that form the foundation of an effective self-marketing strategy; you can then use this strategy to create your own opportunities.

It is important to keep in mind that when you are actively marketing through your résumé and through interview processes, employers may refer to Internet blogs and Web sites such as Facebook (http://www.facebook.com/) and MySpace (http://www.myspace.com) to learn more about you as a potential employee. Go to Google (http://www.google.ca/) and search your name to find out what personal information about you is accessible to potential employers and the general public. Consider the type of information, graphics, and photographs you offer through these sites when you are endeavouring to market your professional attributes.

How Can You Market Yourself?

For students, self-marketing is facilitated by establishing a network, acquiring a mentor, and developing written and verbal communication skills.

Networking and Establishing Support Groups

Establishing a network is a fundamental step in self-marketing. Networking can serve many purposes for students. It involves meeting with a variety of people who share similar interests, who practise in professional areas that are attractive to you, and who can offer new ideas, perspectives, and opportunities. Besides being a valuable way to establish and maintain your sense of professional identity, networking also offers the opportunity to inform others of your interests, activities, and hopes for your future practice.

Networking can produce significant results if you believe in yourself and are committed and prepared to work at it. Be mindful that your networking activities will likely become more focused as you progress in your educational program. Initially, you may feel unsure about the most appropriate place to start to network. In the early years of your program, it may be most beneficial to concentrate your networking activities within your school. As you start to develop some questions and focus related to your career vision, you can benefit from networking resources in the broader community of your health care profession.

Throughout your education, but particularly in its early stages, it is important to discover who your classmates are and how you can establish a sense of involvement in your school. Meeting students at all levels of your program will help you find others with similar goals and interests. It will also offer you the chance to find out about interesting courses, field placement opportunities, and resources, not to mention the support that you can enjoy through your interactions with others who are experiencing similar challenges and adjustments. Becoming actively involved with professional student groups is an excellent way to meet student colleagues and provides many advantages, including the following:

+ The opportunity to meet and work with a large number of faculty members
+ Support in attending local, provincial, national, and possibly international conferences and workshops
+ Opportunities to gain experience in working on committees and in public speaking
+ The development of overall leadership skills

The first step in developing your own network is to make a list of people you think may be helpful to you. Consider all the facets of your life—social, family, school, and work—as you identify potentially helpful people. In addition to student associations, faculty members represent another opportunity for networking that is at your fingertips. Each faculty member has recognized expertise in one or more areas of practice, research, and education. The exchange of interests and ideas can be mutually rewarding for you and the faculty member.

The process of networking with your classmates can be both formal and informal. Joining student groups and committees is one formal means of meeting and working with fellow students. A fourth-year student described the following experience:

> I became active with student groups within 2 months of starting school. From there, things just blossomed until I was making connections with students on a national level through my professional students association. Now that I am ready to graduate and look for a job, I have a network of colleagues I can call on for advice and direction.

Involvement with the student association allowed this student to meet others both from her program and from corresponding programs at other schools. Whether you choose formal settings, informal settings, or both, such involvement means networking with your peers; sharing your vision, goals, and interests with them; and allowing them to keep you in mind during their experiences. You, in turn, can do the same for them as you encounter new experiences.

The exchange of ideas can be a mutually rewarding experience for you and the faculty member. One student reported the following networking experiences in her program school:

> In my final year, I volunteered to be my class representative for student council and also became a member of one of my school's steering committees. These opportunities allowed me to learn more about faculty members and to interact differently with them from the way I would if we were discussing a test grade or paper. The faculty offered guidance, resources, and support.

Another excellent opportunity for networking is provided by volunteer activities. The people you meet while volunteering will help expand your network. Volunteer work is an opportunity to develop new skills and gain experience and insight into a new environment. A good place to start is in your school. Many faculty members and fellow students are involved in committees and organizations and would welcome new ideas, energy, and enthusiasm. Your career vision can also help you identify volunteer activities. For example, if you are interested in working with clients in palliative care, you may consider volunteering in a palliative care unit. The time commitment required for volunteer activities varies, so you need to check whether you can fit outside volunteer activities into your academic schedule without putting undue stress on yourself.

Once you have established your network (or networks), you can target certain individuals and begin to build and maintain a support group. Your support group can consist of fellow students and faculty members who believe in you and want to see you succeed. Surround yourself with individuals who keep a positive attitude and are a source of confidence as you develop an action plan to reach your career goals and, ultimately, your career vision. Seek out those whose feedback you value and whose emotional support you can count on, particularly when you take risks.

You may want to build your support group right now. As you engage in the career planning process, a support group of your peers can help you explore your options and problem-solve as you work with the Model (and network).

Finding a Mentor

The second step in your self-marketing strategy should be to acquire a mentor. A mentor is someone who takes a personal and professional interest in your professional development. Your mentor should be someone with more experience and wisdom who supports and encourages you as you grow and develop in your career (Donner & Wheeler, 2007). Your mentor will guide and support you through all areas of the career planning and development process as you transform your dreams into reality. In the world of health care professionals, mentors generally are experienced individuals who know the ins and outs of the health care environment, know the discipline, have more connections, and have more access to information than less experienced and often younger health care professionals have. Do not restrict yourself to your specific profession or your own professional community when seeking a mentor. Your social and community connections are also excellent resources.

Determine the type of mentor you need and where to find one by reflecting on your career vision and looking at your self-assessment to help you identify exactly the type of help and support you require. Desirable characteristics of any mentor include patience, enthusiasm, knowledge, a sense of humour, and respect (Donner & Wheeler, 2007). Other important considerations when you are determining the fit between you and a potential mentor are the ability of the mentor to be available to you in terms of supporting you to achieve your career goals, the potential mentor's leadership and teaching style, and the willingness of the mentor to commit to the mentoring relationship. This commitment must also be shared by you as the "mentee."

Through coaching and moral support, your mentor can help you scan the environment and can give feedback as you assess your own strengths, identify your career goals, and develop a career plan that fits with your vision. Your mentor can also help you develop your skills in marketing and open doors that will enable you to meet others who can support your career goals and activities (Donner & Wheeler, 2007). Of course, not everyone needs or wants a mentor. However, having a mentor is another valuable way to ensure your career success—so consider it.

A mentor may be a faculty member who has taken a special interest in you, has influenced your career decisions, and has helped open doors for you. You may also encounter professionals in your field placements, summer employment, volunteer activities, and other professional activities who represent role models for you.

Once you have identified a possible mentor, create both informal and formal opportunities for each of you to get to know one another. Such opportunities include volunteer work on similar projects or choosing to sit on a committee of which the mentor is a member.

A fourth-year student described his relationship with a mentor as follows:

> A faculty member from the third year of my program has become an excellent mentor. We have had numerous opportunities to work together, and she has a good idea of my career vision, my strengths, and key areas for my ongoing development. She has provided me with advice and support regarding my career direction, and she has suggested other individuals I could meet with to discuss my interests. I feel that working with a mentor is a great self-marketing strategy that I can continue to use long after I graduate.

Another student described her mentor in the following way:

> She was an influential faculty member who took the time to assist and get to know me. She listened to my vision and identified opportunities for growth and encouraged me to explore them. She provided opportunities for me to be involved both within the school and in the broader professional community. I learned from her professional presentation, and she seemed to take extra time to help me with my professional development.

A senior student described her experience in asking a faculty member to be her mentor as follows:

> I really enjoyed one of my second-year instructors. I often thought that I would like to be just like her when I got to be a "real" professional! I never told her that I admired her; I just assumed she would know that. In my fourth year, she was my advisor for my final field placement. She was still as active and as impressive as I remembered her to be. I decided to tell her that I considered her to be a great professional role model. I also asked her if she would be my mentor. To my surprise, she said that she would be honoured to act as my mentor, and since that meeting, she has met with me to go over my career vision and self-assessment and has already begun to inform me of activities and people she thinks would be helpful to my career.

Developing Your Communication Skills:
Marketing Yourself on Paper

Creating a targeted résumé and other written communication (e.g., business cards) is an important part of self-marketing.

RÉSUMÉS. Your résumé is one of your most valuable written self-marketing strategies. It is a summary of your skills and accomplishments. A résumé is also a way to monitor your progress in building the strengths and expertise that you have identified in your self-assessment.

Creating a résumé requires preparation, patience, practice, practice, and practice! Remember, there is no such thing as a "one size fits all" résumé. You must customize your résumé to ensure that it is effective for each specific opportunity you are pursuing. Use your résumé as a strategic marketing tool to accentuate the accomplishments, skills, and knowledge you identified as part of your self-assessment. You will need to collect some data about a potential field placement or job opportunity before you can customize your résumé. Learn about the organization and the role of students in the organization and in the specific unit, and scan the environment to determine available learning opportunities and how your learning goals may fit with those opportunities.

It is helpful to have a "junk drawer" résumé in which to document all your professional experiences (with a brief description of the skills and accomplishments resulting from each experience), professional and nonprofessional jobs, volunteer activities, extracurricular professional development activities, and professionally related qualifications. Create headings for all categories of activities (i.e., education, awards, field practice experiences, professional activities, professional memberships, employment history, and volunteer activities). If you find that you have headings but no activities to place under them, then you know that one of your career development activities should be related to that area of your professional life. When it is time to submit a résumé, you can create a customized résumé by selecting the information from your "junk drawer" version that is most relevant to the job for which you are applying.

A student résumé has three unique aspects: (1) a list of selected field placements, that is, those placements that provided the opportunity for you to develop the professional competencies of most relevance to the job to which you are applying; (2) a summary of outcome competencies and accomplishments related to field placement experiences; and (3) documentation of past work experiences, including summer and part-time employment.

If your program curriculum includes field placements, it is helpful to provide a list of selected field placements. Include those placement experiences through which you developed and enhanced the professional competencies and knowledge most relevant to the job for which you are applying. Limit the list of selected placements to two or three experiences, focusing on responsibilities, accomplishments, and competencies that relate directly to the advertised professional role.

The field experience summary informs the employer of the scope of practice experiences you have had during your academic career. These experiences can simply be listed; include those you had in the early years of your program and those that provided you with the fundamental knowledge and skills relevant to your discipline. If your program curriculum did not include field placements, include a summary of the strengths you developed during the course of your program.

The components of a student résumé are illustrated in Appendix A.

Your résumé should always be accompanied by a one-page cover letter. The purpose of a cover letter is to encourage the recipient to read your résumé more carefully to determine how your specific learning goals, experience, and abilities fit with his or her organization or society. It should be printed out on personal letterhead paper and attached to your personal business card; together, these will provide all the details the reader needs to get in touch with you. An example of a cover letter can be found in Appendix B.

ELECTRONIC RÉSUMÉS. Bookey-Bassett (2004) notes the significant impact that technology has had on the job search process. Many employers now prefer to receive résumés by e-mail. Electronic résumés can be sent as a Microsoft Word attachment, in a Web portfolio, or on a compact disc (CD) (Bookey-Bassett, 2004; Dixson, 2001; Smith, 1999). Using career portfolios or CD résumés or portfolios allows you to creatively convey your competencies and accomplishments with multimedia technology. Resources for developing electronic résumés can be found in the "Career Planning and Development Resources" section at the end of this guide.

If the employer specifically requests an electronic résumé, determine whether one particular format is required. Copy and paste the résumé into the body of a test e-mail message and send it back to yourself (or to a friend who uses a different e-mail program) to see how the recipient will view your résumé. Keep in mind that when you are applying for a job electronically, a cover letter should accompany your résumé. The letter should be sent in the text portion; send the résumé as an attachment to the e-mail message (Smith, 1999).

BUSINESS CARDS. Business cards provide a simple and professional way to introduce yourself to others and to ensure that they do not forget you. Student business cards need have only the student's name, phone number, and e-mail address. As one student observed:

> I never thought it would be appropriate for students to carry and distribute their own business cards. After a career planning and development workshop, I went home and designed one with a computer program I have. I think this strategy is an effective and creative means of giving others a way to reach me by telephone, fax, or e-mail. I included only my name, the fact that I was a student in my professional program, my university, and contact information. I was encouraged to keep the card simple, and it looks great. Having my own business card also makes me feel more professional.

Another student shared the following:

> Having my own business card makes me feel professional, valued, and significant. I remember when I handed my first business card to a colleague of mine in class. She was very impressed by the professionalism it conveyed. Distributing your own business card not only conveys professionalism but puts the "finishing touch" to the end of an encounter. When done correctly, I think it makes the perfect first and last impression.

Developing Your Communication Skills: Marketing Yourself in Person

Each time you meet someone new, you are presented with a marketing opportunity to accentuate your positive characteristics, take credit for your accomplishments, share your professional goals, and remind others of what you have to contribute. To seize these opportunities effectively, you should rehearse a short self-promotional statement. Then when you meet people and are asked to talk about yourself, you will be ready to clearly, concisely, and confidently articulate your career vision, your current level of knowledge and skills, your present and future career goals, and your unique contributions. You do not need to wait for people to come to you. Become active in your school, student and professional associations, and interest groups, and contribute to an initiative that will help you both build and profile your talents and accomplishments.

INTERVIEWS. Interviews provide another excellent self-marketing opportunity. You will need finely honed interviewing skills whether you are interviewed for a field placement, a job, graduate school, or a volunteer position and whether you are interviewed by a professional association or by a community agency. An interview is a powerful self-marketing opportunity to present your interests, knowledge, skills, and potential in the most positive and appropriate manner.

You should plan for every interview thoughtfully and thoroughly, whether the interview is in application for a field placement, summer job, or health care position. If your career vision, self-assessment, and strategic career plan are up to date and if you have done your preparation, your chances of having a successful interview are good. Your answers to the interview questions can demonstrate that you have relevant interests, entry skills, knowledge, and (most important) the enthusiasm and ability to learn and make contributions to the organization. The interview also gives you an opportunity to have your questions answered so that if you are offered the position, you can consult with your mentor and professional colleagues to make a well-informed decision about whether the position is the right one for you.

Some individuals find it helpful to audiotape or videotape themselves in a mock interview so that they can identify their strengths and the areas they would like to improve on prior to experiencing the "real thing." Ask a student colleague to help you with this exercise and offer you some feedback. Your mentor is another excellent resource for practising your interview skills.

JUSTINE In preparation for an interview at a field placement organization, Justine obtained (1) copies of the philosophy statements of the specific discipline's department and the unit to which she was applying, (2) a copy of the hospital's strategic plan and job description of the field practice area, and (3) a schedule of selected professional development opportunities she could take advantage of as a student in the organization. She then spoke with two students who had experience in that organization. Finally, she met with her mentor to discuss how the skills and accomplishments identified in her self-assessment and her related learning goals fit with the available learning opportunities and with the philosophies and plans of the department and organization. Justine also participated in a mock interview with her mentor before her actual interview. Justine would use this same process to prepare for a job interview.

REFERENCES. Faculty members, mentors, field practice preceptors, part-time and summer job employers, and contacts from volunteer activities can be appropriate sources of references for students. It is important that you select as referees individuals who are familiar with your current level of professional skill development and recent accomplishments relevant to the practice area to which you are applying. If a referee is not knowledgeable about your recent work, provide him or her with a copy of your résumé and any other information that supports your application for the job (e.g., vision, self-assessment, strategic career plan, or field placement evaluations)

It is important to ask potential referees well in advance if they would be willing to provide a positive reference for you. After a job interview, offer the names of your referees if you would like to pursue employment with that organization. Contact your referees each time you give their name as a reference. Inform them of the specific requirements of the job you are seeking, and give them any other information that will help them provide a comprehensive reference. Be sure that each referee has a copy of the résumé you submitted and any new information that may not appear on your résumé.

Self-marketing is about using all your resources to present yourself in the strongest and most positive way. Remember that the most important resource you have for shaping your own future is you! Keep your career vision and goals in mind. Creating an effective self-marketing strategy takes time, effort, and patience. Following these strategies will contribute to realizing your goals. The following excerpt summarizes Justine's thoughts on the process of career planning:

> Learning about the career planning process motivated me to think more seriously about my career plans and what I have done and need to do to accomplish them. I have realized the need to clarify my plans and put them into action through a number of realistic self-marketing strategies. This experience has allowed me to be more self-directed and actively involved. I believe I have a better understanding of the numerous opportunities available to me and how I can take advantage of them in an effective way.

Complete Activity 6 to assess your marketing readiness.

Activity (6) Marketing Yourself

Self-marketing is representing yourself in the best way possible by using all your resources.

➢ How is your marketing readiness? Use the following checklist to answer that question.

- ❑ I have a career vision.
- ❑ I know my environment.
- ❑ I know myself.
- ❑ I know I am my best marketer.
- ❑ I know how to network.
- ❑ I have a support group.
- ❑ I have a mentor.
- ❑ I have a current résumé.
- ❑ I have a business card.
- ❑ I have excellent interview skills.

➢ Which areas need some attention? Develop a plan to meet those needs.

What I Need To Do	When I Will Do It
1.	1.
2.	2.
3.	3.
4.	4.
5.	5.

What Have You Accomplished?

Congratulations! You have made your first tour through the Donner-Wheeler Career Planning and Development Model. You have learned how you can use your dreams, your environment, your self-knowledge, and your career plan to explore how you can influence your educational activities to achieve your current and future career goals. You will return to the Model again and again as you build your health care career. We hope it serves you well!

WHAT NEXT?

Career planning and development is a continuous process—a "work-in-progress." To ensure that you are getting the most from your career planning activities, you should consider an overall evaluation of how it is working for you. Complete the following questionnaire at each transition time in your academic program (e.g., at the middle and end of each term, at the completion of a field placement experience, or at evaluation meetings) and on an annual basis. It will help you determine which phases of the Model need more attention, need updating, or need more consultation and support. You can also use your journal as an ongoing record of how you are moving forward as a student, as a future health care professional, and as a person.

How Am I Doing?

Visioning

❑ I can describe my ideal vision for my future.

Scanning

❑ I am aware of the current realities and future trends at the school, local, and national levels, both in health care and in my profession.

Assessing

❑ I can describe my strengths.

❑ I can describe key areas for development.

❑ I know how others would describe me.

❑ My current academic activities are a good match with my values, beliefs, knowledge, skills, interests, and vision.

Planning

❑ I can identify my career vision and my short- and long-term career goals.

❑ I have a written career development plan in place.

❑ I know what steps to take over the next 3 to 6 months to further my progress toward my career vision.

Marketing

❑ I have established a relevant network.

❑ I have acquired a mentor or am considering acquiring one.

❑ I continue to develop my communication skills.

❑ I have an up-to-date résumé.

Choosing Your First Job as a Health Care Professional

Congratulations on successfully completing your professional program! You have worked hard to achieve your health profession degree. The possibilities are endless, but excitement can be accompanied by anxiety. You have some important decisions to make. Using the Model to guide your exploration and assessment of job opportunities can give you a sense of control and confidence regarding your decision making. Many students ask the following questions:

+ How can I make sure that I am choosing the job that is right for me?
+ How can I sort out the benefits of one job offer compared with another?
+ What types of questions should I be asking?

You are now ready to use the Donner-Wheeler Career Planning and Development Model to help position you to get the job you want. It is important to return to each phase of the Model as you embark on the exciting process of choosing your first position as a health care professional.

YOUR CAREER VISION

Time to dream again! This is an exciting moment in your personal and professional life. How have you envisioned yourself as a professional in your field? Use your vision to guide your choice of where to submit your job applications. How do the positions to which you are applying fit with your vision? Can you see the potential of the positions to help you actualize your vision? Your vision can help you make choices that fit with your current interests, needs, knowledge, and dreams.

YOUR ENVIRONMENTAL SCAN

As you prepare to move into the workplace, it is important to update your environmental scan. Include a scan of national, provincial, and local issues and trends. The purpose of this scan is two-fold: (1) to determine the issues and trends in your particular area of interest and focus, and (2) to become aware of the current realities in both the profession and the health care system in general. Knowledge of what is currently happening in your area of interest will help you get a sense of what is "out there" in terms of specific jobs, issues and gaps in those job opportunities, and practice challenges you might be able to anticipate and reflect on as you revisit your self-assessment. An awareness of issues and trends in the profession as well as in the health care system in general will serve you well in the interview process. Your scan could also include enhancing your awareness of general employability skills. (For example, the Conference Board of Canada Employability Skills 2000+ list is a list of employability skills that can expand your self-assessment and scanning activities; go to http://www.conferenceboard.ca/education/learning-tools/pdfs/esp2000.pdf to view the skills list). With this knowledge, you can feel confident responding to potential questions focused on what you see as current and future issues for health care professionals entering the workforce at this time. The scan can also cue you about questions you might like to ask in an interview.

If you know the agency to which you are applying, a significant focus of your scan should be on learning about the mandate, philosophy, and resources of your discipline's department. Obtain a copy of the job description to determine how your skills, knowledge, and interests fit with the job requirements and how to market those qualities. Your scan will also help you determine if the supports, resources, and culture of a given organization fit with your vision and values. It is also important to assess the degree to which organizations acknowledge and respond to the unique challenges experienced by new graduates as they make the transition from students to employees.

YOUR SELF-ASSESSMENT

Return to your self-assessment. This will not be the last time you do a self-assessment, but this is the one time that doing it will serve as a springboard to your first position as a health care professional. Complete this self-assessment with a focus on your values, interests, knowledge, and skills related to your particular career vision. If you do not have one area of interest, complete your assessment with a view to consolidating your overall professional interests, skills, and knowledge base. As you apply for specific jobs, you can refine your assessment to reflect the particular position at hand. In essence, you are streamlining your self-assessment to help you target the position you wish to secure. The position should also allow you to continue to advance toward your career vision. Undoubtedly, the process of completing your assessment will remind you of all that you have learned and of your identity as a unique professional who has much to contribute to the workplace.

YOUR STRATEGIC CAREER PLAN

Your strategic career plan can be focused on short-term and long-term goals related to getting the job you want. Your scan has given you important information about opportunities and realities; your assessment has clarified your current interests, skills, knowledge, and values; and your vision is your future. Using this information as your guide, ask yourself what you need to do to meet your short-term and long-term goals and who can help you. You can focus your activities on getting more information, contacting resources, developing your résumé, or preparing for an interview.

MARKETING

Make an appointment with your mentor to discuss your graduation plans. Bring your mentor up to date with your vision and career-planning activities, and seek specific support to help you assess the relative merits of job opportunities. Your mentor can also assist you as you develop your strategic career plan.

Information from health care organizations can help you determine the fit between your vision, interests, and skills and the goals and philosophies of individual settings. You can collect much of this information long before the interview stage to decide whether you want to consider a particular agency for future employment.

When you select agencies for potential employment, you need to customize your résumé for each employer. Review the résumé section in Chapter 2 as well as Appendix A for tips on résumé development.

You *have* the knowledge you need to select the job that best matches your interests and your vision. You are in the driver's seat; enjoy the ride!

4

Do You Need More Help?

You have covered a lot of material. If it seems overwhelming or if you are not sure you have a good understanding of it, your first step should be to go back to the beginning of this guide and review the material and activities. Then look at the references provided in the "Career Planning and Development Resources" section at the end of the guide. You can also join or establish a support group with student peers who are also using this guide to help with their career planning experience. Sharing your questions, ideas, and strategies can provide you with relevant support and new resources. Career resources at your college or university and faculty members with an interest in career development are other supports available to you. The Internet is another valuable resource. You probably already use it a great deal to enhance your education, but consider using it to find resources to help you manage your student career and make sound decisions about your future career. Of course, there are also student and professional organizations that provide many paths to pursue learning and professional growth. Armed with a clear understanding of who you are and what you want to contribute to your discipline, you will be ready for that future.

Alone we can do so little, but together we can achieve so much.

– Helen Keller

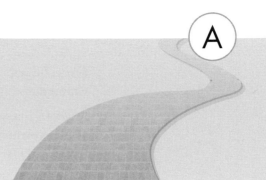

Student Résumés

Generic Student Résumé

The broad health profession competencies included in this generic résumé can be replaced with discipline-specific language and competencies. Examples of the type of information you can include in your student résumé are also included for your reference.

Name
123 Four Street
City, Province/State Postal/Zip code
Tel: H: (123) 456-7891
E-mail: j3smity@coldmail.com
Fax: (123) 456-7890

Career Objective: (To obtain an entry-level position in X department, where I can continue to advance my knowledge and skills in Y and collaborate with colleagues and clients to achieve a high quality of care.)

EDUCATION

> Degree
> Name of University
> City, Province/State
> Anticipated date of completion (month, year)

HONOURS AND AWARDS

> Member, University/Professional Honour Society
> Faculty Dean's List
> School/Program Student Leadership Award

SELECTED FIELD EXPERIENCES

> **Student, Second Year, Rehabilitation Unit**
> Worked collaboratively within a team model to provide comprehensive care to adults in the stroke rehabilitation unit. Acknowledged for effective communication skills with clients and interdiscipli-

---

Continued

nary colleagues, health-related client teaching, and leadership skills within the scope of student role.

Acquired Competencies: Basic assessment and intervention skills, active student member of health care team, therapeutic communication skills.

Student, Third Year, Community Clinic
Worked effectively with preceptor in providing comprehensive family-centred care. Acknowledged for strong communication skills with clients across the lifespan and effective psychosocial care. Contributed to interdisciplinary client care discussions.

Acquired Competencies: Positive therapeutic communication skills, health teaching, family-centred care, discharge planning.

PROFESSIONAL ACTIVITIES

Year	Second-year representative at school council
Year	First-year representative at school council

PROFESSIONAL MEMBERSHIPS

Student member, professional association

EMPLOYMENT HISTORY

Month, year–
  present

Salesperson
Part-time position
Required to work independently, providing supervision and training to new salespersons. Responsible for meeting consumer needs in a professional manner. Utilized effective organizational and management skills. Collaborative member of sales team.

Months, year

Personal Care Assistant
Summer employment
Required to work independently, providing basic care to residents. Utilized positive and effective communication skills. Acknowledged for strengths in conveying compassion, sensitivity, and respect to residents and families. Reliable and responsible.

COMMUNITY AND VOLUNTEER ACTIVITIES:

(Include experiences that are relevant to the type of work you are seeking. It is helpful to include volunteer experiences that have afforded you the opportunity to further enhance competencies necessary for your professional practice or to develop new competencies that will add to your practice.)

Months, year

Volunteer, Canadian Cancer Society
Canvasser

Résumé of a Graduating Student Seeking First Health Care Position in a Mental Health Care Setting

The broad health care professional competencies included in this generic résumé can be replaced with discipline-specific language and competencies. If your program curriculum did not include field placements, include a summary of your strengths in your résumé.

Name
1111 Twelve Street
City, Province/State Postal/Zip code
H (444) 222-3333
E-mail: donovan@nomail.com
Fax: (444) 777-8888

Career Objective: To secure an entry-level position in the mental health care area, where I can further develop my professional practice competencies and contribute my growing strengths in communication and interdisciplinary teamwork.

Summary of Strengths (optional): Over the course of my academic program, I have created and taken advantage of opportunities to develop strengths in client advocacy, health teaching, family-centred care, professional and therapeutic communication, and essential competencies of practice. I am a self-directed, inquisitive individual who enjoys challenge and is committed to being an active and contributing member of my profession.

EDUCATION

Year–present   Degree

           Name of University
           City, Province/State
           Anticipated date of completion: May 2003

HONOURS AND AWARDS

1999–2000   Dean's List

SELECTED FIELD EXPERIENCES

Student, 4th Year, City Mental Health Outpatient Unit
Young adult and adolescent client groups.
With preceptor, co-facilitated psychoeducational groups for newly diagnosed young adults and adolescents with schizophrenia.
Provided individualized client and family education related to illness and medication.

Continued

Acquired Competencies: Administration of Mini-Mental State Examination, with supervision; facilitation of support and psycho-educational groups; individual supportive counselling.

Accomplishments: Developed an educational pamphlet targeting young adults and adolescents.

Student, 3rd Year, Community Outreach Program
Collaborated with interdisciplinary team to provide support to older adults living alone after discharge from hospital.

Acquired Competencies: Gained skills in engaging the older adult client, assessing health needs within the context of the individual's lifestyle, and managing issues related to treatment adherence.

Accomplishments: Acknowledged for strengths in developing a positive rapport with hard-to-reach clients and in adapting care to the community setting.

OTHER FIELD EXPERIENCES

Year, name of organization, and focus of experience
Year, name of organization, and focus of experience

PROFESSIONAL ACTIVITIES

Year(s)   Vice-president of program's student association
Year(s)   Year representative for school council

PROFESSIONAL MEMBERSHIPS

Professional association
Student group
Community mental health group

EMPLOYMENT HISTORY

Year(s)   **Assistant**
Summer employment, long-term care facility, city
Developed skills in teamwork, organization, communication with individuals who have difficulty with expressive and receptive communication, and working as a member of a health care team.

Accomplishments: Organized a family support picnic for residents and families.

Continued

Year(s)	**Waiter**
	Restaurant, city
	Developed skills in organization, time management, and consumer-focused service.
	Provided competent and professional service to restaurant patrons.
	Reliable and responsible.

COMMUNITY AND VOLUNTEER ACTIVITIES

(Include experiences that are relevant to the type of work you are seeking. It is helpful to include volunteer experiences that have afforded you the opportunity to further enhance competencies necessary to your professional practice or to develop new competencies that will add to your practice.)

Year(s)	Continue to organize annual family support picnics for residents of a long-term care facility and their families.

Graduating Student Cover Letter

9999 90th Ave.
City, province/state
Postal/zip code

Date

Ms. Jane Smith
Program Director
(Program name)
Metropolitan Health Centre
(City, Province/State, postal/zip code)

Dear Ms. Smith:

I am writing in response to the advertisement posted on the Human Resources bulletin board for the xxxxx position in the xxxxx Program.

I will be graduating from my xxxxx program in month, year. Over the course of my education, I have endeavoured to develop a wide range of professional practice competencies relevant to the field of xxxxx. I have taken advantage of many learning opportunities, with the goal of achieving strengths in therapeutic communication, assessment, intervention, and interdisciplinary teamwork. I believe I have been successful in obtaining a solid foundation in xxxxx practice. I would look forward to continuing my professional development in this area of practice in your program.

The enclosed résumé has more details about how my professional practice and other academic experiences have prepared me to fulfill the needs of your xxxxx position. I would be delighted to discuss my potential contribution to your program and look forward to hearing from you.

Yours truly,

(Signature)

(Name)

Enclosure: Résumé

Career Planning and Development Resources: A Selected Reading List

> **TIP:** Check your local bookstore or library for current career planning and development resources. The shelves are full. The following are good "reads" from our bookshelves.

BOOKS AND JOURNAL ARTICLES

Beatty, R. (2003). *The interview kit.* New York: John Wiley.

Beatty, R. (2003). *The resume kit.* New York: John Wiley.

Bolles, R. N. (2008). *What color is your parachute? A practical manual for job-hunters and career-changers.* Berkeley, CA: Ten Speed Press.

Bookey-Basset, S. (2004). Marketing yourself. In G. J. Donner & M. M. Wheeler (Eds.), *Taking control of your nursing career* (2nd ed., pp. 63–90). Toronto, ON: Elsevier.

Covey, S. (1989). *The seven habits of highly effective people.* New York: Simon & Schuster.

Darling, D. (2003). *The networking survival guide: Get the success you want by tapping into the people you know.* New York: McGraw-Hill.

Dikel, M., & Roehm, F. (2006). *Guide to internet job searching.* New York: McGraw-Hill.

Dixson, K. (2001). Every job searcher needs an e-resume. *Career Planning and Adult Development Journal, 17*(4), 66–78.

Donner, G., & Wheeler, M. (Eds.). (2004). *Taking control of your nursing career* (2nd ed.). Toronto, ON: Elsevier.

Donner, G., & Wheeler, M. (2007). *A guide to coaching and mentoring in nursing.* Geneva, Switzerland: International Council of Nurses.

Donner, G. & Wheeler, M. (In press). *Taking control of your career: A handbook for health professionals.* Toronto, ON: Elsevier.

Handy, C. (2005). *Understanding organizations*. New York: Penguin Global.

Ittelson, J. C. (2001). Building an e-identity for each student. *EDUCAUSE Quarterly, 24*(4).

Krannich, R., & Enelow, W. (2002). *Best resumes and CVs for international jobs*. Lynchburg, VA: Career Masters Institutes.

Miller, T. (2003). *Building and managing a career in nursing: Strategies for advancing your career*. Indianapolis, IN: Sigma Theta Tau International.

Moses, B. (2000). *The good news about careers: How you'll be working in the next decade*. New York: Jossey-Bass.

Rath, T. (2007). *Strengths finder 2.0*. New York: Gallup Press.

Schein, E. (1990). *Discovering your real values* (2nd ed.). San Francisco: Pfeiffer & Co.

Schein, E. (2006). *Career anchors: Self-assessment*. San Francisco: John Wiley & Sons.

Simonsen, P. (2000). *Career compass: Navigating your career strategically in the new century*. Palo Alto, CA: Davies-Black.

Smith, R. (1999). *Electronic resumes and online networking*. Franklin Lakes, NJ: Career Press.

Vallano, A. (2002). *Your career in nursing: Manage your future in the new world of health care*. New York: Simon & Schuster.

Verma, S., Paterson, M., & Medves, J. (2006). Core competencies for health care professionals. *Journal of Allied Health, 35*(2), 109–115.

Waddell, J., Donner, G. J., & Wheeler, M. M. (2009). *Building your nursing career: A guide for students* (3rd ed.). Toronto, ON: Elsevier.

Wood, M. J., & Ross-Kerr, J. C. (2003). *Canadian nursing: Issues and perspectives* (4th ed.). Toronto, ON: Elsevier.

ONLINE RESOURCES

Electronic Portfolios

- Abrenica, Y. *Using electronic portfolios*. Retrieved May 7, 2008, from San Diego State University Web site: http://edweb.sdsu.edu/courses/edtec596r/students/Abrenica/Abrenica.html
- Lorenzo, G., & Ittelson, J. (2005). *An overview of e-portfolios*. Retrieved May 7, 2008, from The EDUCAUSE Learning Initiative Web site: http://www.educause.edu/ir/library/pdf/ELI3001.pdf

Employability Skills

- *The Conference Board of Canada employability skills.* Retrieved May 8, 2008, from http://www.calsca.com/conference_board.htm

Values Clarification

- Mensing, S. *Tips on values clarification.* Retrieved May 8, 2008, from http://www.emoclear.com/processes/values.html
- Possible values clarification exercises. (from *Instructor's resource manual for freshman orientation course*). Retrieved May 8, 2008, from Middle Tennessee State University Web site: http://mtsu.edu/~u101irm/valuesex.html